Learning to Live Rest and Let Go

A psychiatrist's handbook on resting effectively in order to stop worrying and manage stress

FERNANDO SARRÁIS

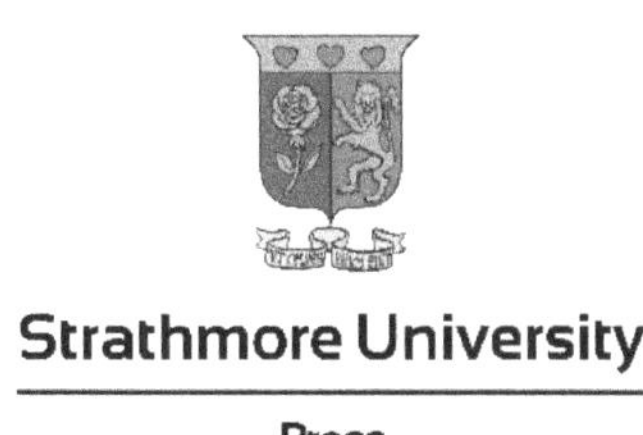

Strathmore University
Press

The original Spanish edition was first published in 2011 by Ediciones Universidad de Navarra, S.A. (EUNSA), Pamplona, Spain under the Person and Culture Collection (No. 2).

SUP acknowledges the permission granted it by Dr. Fernando Sarráis and by EUNSA to translate and publish the book in English. Strathmore University Press (SUP) appreciates the enormous effort of Martyn Drakard who translated the book from Spanish into English. SUP also acknowledges the proof-reading work of the English manuscript carried out by Andrea Kaggwa, Fr Joe Barbendrier and Joakim Mwamba.

Cover page design and layout by Jotham Njoroge

Published by Strathmore University Press

ISBN: 9789966054302

PREFACE TO THE ENGLISH EDITION

Modern times have seen the loss of a proper understanding of rest as most people are overly concerned about professional and social progress to which they dedicate most of their time. Little time is set aside for meaningful physical and psychological rest which is necessary for a healthy mind and body. Modern times have also seen a misunderstanding of rest where it is viewed as wasting time or even worse, doing nothing.

Rest is a time for a person to ease out of daily worries and cares which may impede efficient functioning at work, home and other social environments. Rest does not mean that the causes of a person's daily worries and cares will disappear, but it helps a person to refresh so as to be more sober in facing those worries and cares.

Everyone, old or young is in need of meaningful rest and hence restful activities and moments should be an integral part of human life. Human beings are not mechanical instruments or machines and hence rest should be incorporated into a person's daily routine: in any case, machines too need some oiling and greasing and checkups to improve on performance. Taking care of the way a person rests results in a happier and more fruitful life.

The translation of this book into English was provoked by the realization that there are many people in Kenya and East Africa who are experiencing the three illnesses which the author cites as being prevalent in the West: *burn-out*, nerve and muscle pains and chronic weakness. The author points out that these *psychosomatic* illnesses have at their root chronic psychological tension which is due to lack of rest and relaxation. The illnesses according to Dr Sarrais occur in people who tend to be perfectionist, extremely responsible and who make heavy demands on themselves. This book has been written for such people who least know how to rest and consequently are always in a state of tension. This continuous state of tension is the result of such peoples "pathological need to fulfil their obligations, while abandoning the duty they have towards themselves: namely, rest, relaxation and knowing how to enjoy life."

There are many ways of resting and in this book the author gives ideas of rest. Additionally, the author also points out to the reader various things that render our bodies tired and fatigued. Many people interpret the signs their bodies give them wrongly and end up putting more pressure on themselves. For example, when one is dozing while working, it means one hasn't given attention to their sleep and this could end up crippling the work output. Many of these aspects have been dealt with in the book and will help you know how to rest better and make the best out of life.

Dr. Peter Kwenjera
Narobi, 1st July 2020

CONTENTS

1 INTRODUCING REST

"And on the seventh day God finished his work which he had done; and he rested on the seventh day from all his work which he had done" (Genesis 2:2)

This book is the fruit of many years of professional dedication to treating physical and psychological problems related to stress and anxiety, caused by excess work or having to meet deadlines, without taking time off to relax and recover one's energies. In other words, the problems derived from an imbalance between tiredness and rest.

My main purpose is *to show how to prevent psychological fatigue* (both emotional and intellectual), especially the tiredness that accumulates over time and ends up becoming chronic. This kind of tiredness passes unnoticed for years, and is not easy to treat. Physical tiredness, however, is easy to detect and remedy.

In these pages certain ideas are repeated time and again, like the catchy words of a song:

- That psychological tiredness is related to lifestyle;
- That it produces negative feelings, such as fear, anxiety, worry, sadness, rushing around, and
- That rest depends on a few activities that stimulate positive feelings and cancel out the negative ones.

By repeating I aim to impress in the reader's mind the main point of the book, and from time to time will also use popular sayings.

Since the book *is meant for the general reader*, and not the specialist, it may lack academic depth, but it makes up for this by being accessible to the majority of readers who experience this imbalance between tiredness and rest.

I spend much time explaining to my patients how not to get so tired and learn how to rest more and better. This little book can spare me some of that time; it will be a welcome companion to the medical prescriptions patients often have to take home.

I did not write the book to be read quickly or at a go, but slowly so it can be thought about, even read again or at least certain parts of it.

It is intended to prevent rather than cure, and does not recommend specific treatments for physical or psychological changes related to chronic tiredness.

***

Many people focus all their attention on what they have to do in the world outside themselves: work, family, friends, trying to do it all well, at the best possible time, and making everyone happy. But they pay little attention to their inner world, their physical needs and, above all, their psychological and spiritual needs. These people know how to take good care of other people, *but not of themselves.*

Often, as the years go by, when they have less stamina due to age, they start to show signs and symptoms of chronic fatigue which, in many cases, affects their bodies in the form of severe headaches, asthenia (general weakness), insomnia, back pains, digestive problems, skin diseases, high blood pressure, etc. They go to the family doctor or a specialist for a solution so they can continue working at the same pace as before. But they are quite unaware of the relationship between these bodily symptoms and the chronic stress they have lived with for many years, and which has produced a general and chronic wear and tear. They do not look for a solution for the cause, but for the symptoms, and so their condition is usually irreversible. These people go from one medical test and check-up to the next and receive treatment and take medication for years without solving the root problem. With time, psychological complications develop, ending in depression. I always tell my patients: "After tension comes depression".

To make the point abundantly clear regarding the dangerous imbalance between tiredness and recovery, tension and relaxation, activity and rest, I will mention three physical illnesses that are "in fashion" in the West (and not only in the West): burn-out; nerve and muscle pains and chronic weakness. These and other illnesses grouped under the heading of *psychosomatic* have at their root psychological tension, which has become chronic due to lack of rest and relaxation. They occur in people who tend to be perfectionist, extremely responsible, who make heavy demands on themselves, and are result and success-oriented; workaholics, people who easily become obsessed, who have to be in control of every situation, who feel guilty if things are not working out, and highly competitive to the point of excess. They are always in a state of tension, owing to their pathological need to fulfil their obligations, while abandoning the duty they have towards themselves: namely, rest, relaxation and knowing how to enjoy life.

This book is written especially for people like these because they are the ones who least know how to rest.

2 TIREDNESS AND ITS CONSEQUENCES

I already mentioned in the introduction some of the consequences of tiredness, especially chronic tiredness. As a psychiatrist I will concentrate on its psychological aspect.

I will leave to physiologists and biochemists its organic manifestations, those related to the production and breakdown of chemical substances that activate and inhibit the brain and the nervous system. I will also leave to the internists those sensations of tiredness that accompany certain physical illnesses; such sensations are properly called *asthenia,* one symptom more of these illnesses. Asthenia appears also in infections, anemia, hypothyroidism, myopathies, liver diseases such as hepatitis, the ingestion of certain drugs (*e.g.* chemotherapy) and intestinal malabsorption.

To distinguish non-organic tiredness from the tiredness caused by physical illness, one needs to look for other symptoms that go together with asthenia in organic illnesses. To treat this kind of tiredness or organic asthenia is to treat its cause, organic illness. An organic cause of tiredness is to be suspected when the patient has neither carried out nor is carrying out presently some activity that can explain his tiredness.

I also leave to moralists the question of spiritual fatigue or acedia, which has to do with the spiritual aspect of human beings.

When someone is tired from having kept up a physical or intellectual activity without a break, his *performance and efficiency* decrease in inverse proportion to his increased tiredness.

Certain psychic warnings begin to appear associated with malaise and suffering (tiredness is one of them), such as irritability, interior restlessness, anxiety (even anguish), and the tendency to avoid situations where special effort is required.

When he can take no more, the patient can feel the urge and the need to get involved in *inappropriate activities* in order to "escape" or counteract his malaise and restlessness immediately, in such things as excessive consumption of alcohol, sweets and chocolate; pornographic books and magazines or videos, drugs and other stimulants. Or in other things such as serious gambling and anything that attracts attention, such as compulsive spending, etc. to distract from what makes him tired and bored.

Besides, since people with chronic tiredness have used up all their vital energy, or better said, worn it down, they have less will power to do what they should and avoid doing what they should not do; in short, less self-control. Instead, they have a greater facility to become "addicts' of either something that continues wearing them out (like running straight into the arms of the enemy) or that helps them escape their tiredness.

The tendency to escape from what makes them tired and their reduced will power and self-control lead them into harmful addictions, causing frustration and dissatisfaction, pushing them still further into the wrong kind of escape. This creates a dangerous *vicious circle*: tiredness-escape-addiction-frustration-escape.

When the tiredness is excessive, their physical and psychological functions diminish. They have less capacity for concentration and paying attention, thought processes slow down, and there is greater difficulty in connecting ideas and reaching conclusions. They can sit facing a problem for a long time, unable to solve it. Their decision-making capacity is also affected and they cannot see clearly the right path to take. They are filled with doubts, which makes them anxious and restless since they find it hard to go ahead with their usual tasks and complete them, and so be able to rest from them.

2.1 Reduction of will-power

Less energy and will-power is evident in their inability to perform any task that requires effort or is a little complicated. This inability goes together with a feeling of emotional denial. They let time pass without fulfilling their obligations and allowing jobs to pile up, even ones that are easy to do such as putting personal items in order, making a phone call, or buying something they need.

With so little energy and will-power, everything seems to be enormously difficult and impossible to carry out, from getting up, bathing and dressing and preparing breakfast to those things they used to like doing before, like sport, reading, music, etc. Unless a person rests, this can continue until he just cannot go on anymore.

For some people, particularly young people, lack of will-power can be due to too little physical exercise (lack of fortitude), as happens with lazy, easy-going types who deliberately avoid any kind of effort and let themselves be carried along by what they feel like. Such people say they always feel tired and lethargic. Sometimes they are just making excuses for not doing what they should or what others ask them to do, because they do only what they feel like doing. But other times, it is a case of genuine tiredness, which may be due to their not doing anything useful or satisfying (something that makes them feel good, which helps them rest psychologically), or to doing only what their feelings tell them are good for them (which develops their emotional state but is not good for their will-power).

To help people distinguish if their tiredness is real (*e.g.* because of prolonged effort) or false (because of doing nothing and being bored), it is enough to find out what they have been doing in the past few days: if nothing that required intense and continued effort, then it must be tiredness of the second type.

To treat the *tiredness of the lazy, easygoing person*, it is necessary to follow a gradual plan of recovery of the will-power, including a daily schedule of activities that require personal effort. The plan should be supervised by experienced, older people with a certain moral authority over the person who is developing his will-power.

2.2 Anaesthetizing the affectivity (emotions and attitudes)

From the affective point of view, tiredness is evident from a reduced attraction for pleasant things, which is a kind of anesthesia of the affectivity, which leads to *anhedonia* (inability to find joy or pleasure in activities one usually enjoys). Also common is the presence of an emotional hypersensitivity with what is unpleasant; this is manifested when almost all the ambient stimuli produce distaste, irritability and frustration, and make a person escape and isolate himself to get a feeling of relief. This is not the solution, however, because the problem, which is tiredness, continues inside him wherever he goes.

The lack of emotional vibration leads over time to loss of interest in things and people, to sadness and anguish because a person finds no meaning in his daily existence; all of these are symptoms of a *depression,* the common complication of chronically tired people.

3 REST AND ITS CONSEQUENCES

It is obvious that if the after-effects of tiredness are negative and unpleasant, the after-effects of rest are positive since rest relieves or suppresses the effects of tiredness. This is similar to what happens when one has a need (to eat, drink or sleep). When the need is satisfied, one notices a relief from the negative sensations that came with the need.

Some people who are very outgoing but lacking self-knowledge know very well the work they have to do, how to do it to be successful and make others happy, but they are *unable to detect their own feelings of tiredness* until the physical and psychological symptoms start to appear.

Even then they do not seek help because they do not relate the symptoms with the cause, chronic tiredness. And if they do seek help, they refuse to accept the explanation of a specialist and the need to rest. Obviously unless such people learn to know themselves better, they will fare badly because once they feel relieved of the symptoms they will get very tired again and rest little, and collapse again. In these cases, someone close to the person concerned has to feel responsible to shield him from excess of tiredness and push him to rest and relax.

Sometimes it is enough to stop doing what makes us tired in order to rest. Other times, it will be necessary to do specific things that help rest. Some kinds of activities help anyone to rest, (such as lying down, relaxing, sleeping, doing physical exercise). Other activities help certain people rest, such as playing an instrument, painting, fishing, watching sports matches, hunting and fishing, etc). They are activities one has done often which make him feel good and produce positive feelings like joy, relaxation, excitement and enthusiasm.

Generally, we rest with activities that help us enjoy ourselves thoroughly and produce no negative emotions (*e.g.* of guilt) once they are over, as happens with activities that give us pleasure but go against our moral conscience because they are neither proper nor good.

Sometimes the tiredness can be so intense that a person is unable to do anything, even those things that used to help him rest. In such cases of extreme exhaustion, one should stop doing what makes him tired and wait for the physical and psychological energy to come back, allowing him to do what he enjoys doing so he can rest.

3.1 Preventing exhaustion

In cases of extreme tiredness or exhaustion, it is important for the person to learn why and how he arrived at that situation, and to firmly resolve not to let himself get so tired again; besides dealing with tiredness at that time, one should prevent future occurrences.

Prevention is possible by keeping a balance day by day between tiredness and rest, between activities that consume energy and those that restore it. *Every day we must enjoy ourselves because every day we suffer; every day we must relax because every day we become tense.* With practice we can manage to achieve this balance until it becomes automatic, as happens with many other habits. And so one's quality of life improves and the pathological after-effects of habitual deep-seated tiredness are prevented.

3.2 Rest is a duty

Many people learn from childhood how to work hard, to fulfil their obligations, be responsible, serious, and demanding on themselves, but they do not know how to relax physically and psychologically, to enjoy themselves, how to say "Enough!", or "Later" or "No", and they become slaves of *the high demands they make on themselves*; and to such an extent that even when they are resting they have strong feelings of guilt because they think they are being selfish or idle, and straightaway put a stop to their rest. They may even decide to avoid rest in future, associating it with that unpleasant feeling of guilt. They do not realize that if they are to work well they have to rest, because one can be tired and working away, even for years, but the quality of the work will suffer. Not only that, sufficient rest prolongs one's years of effective professional work since one avoids psychological illnesses which very often lead to situations of temporary unemployment and even being permanently unfit for work.

Those people who become so engrossed in work and useful activities must convince themselves that "rest" (dedicating time to enjoyable activities) is a *duty*, one more necessary occupation like eating, sleeping or showering and dressing. If they think of rest as a duty they will no longer feel guilty when they change their routine and try to fit in a healthy balance between work and rest. Once they succeed and see the improvement physically and psychologically, they will realize how useful it is and will be motivated to keep it up.

3.3 Positive effects of physical and psychological rest

Physical rest has various positive effects as it produces a sensation of greater energy, vitality and physical well-being. It is also accompanied by an emotional reaction of lightheartedness and joy. This reaction makes one more optimistic, quick-witted and clear-headed. Physical rest moves the will to make fresh plans and carry them out in the belief that they are quite possible and within one's reach.

What earlier, in one's state of tiredness, seemed impossible now looks easy and sure of success.

The effect of physical tiredness is due to *biochemical and physiological changes* (changes in the hormonal levels and the neurotransmitters in the brain). These changes affect one's emotional state through the limbic system, in such a way that

- The negative emotions and feelings that go with tiredness disappear
- Positive emotions emerge which favour and stimulate the proper working of the intellect and the will
- They go together with a physical sensation of energy and vitality enabling one to do more and do better the things that have to be done.

And so the Latin saying *mens sana in corpore sano* (a healthy mind in a healthy body) becomes real in one's daily life.

Psychological rest, owing to the psychosomatic unity of the human being, produces positive *physical effects* as well as the *psychological effects* already mentioned. In the next sections we shall deal with this two-way psychosomatic correlation.

4 PHYSICAL REST

Everyone has his own way of resting his body, but I shall concentrate on three general ways: restfulness, sleeping and relaxation. The three overlap and interact with one another.

4.1. Restfulness

The verb "to be resting", which is synonymous with "to rest" has several meanings, but the most interesting for us is this: "for something or someone to remain in a state of calm and stillness". Physical stillness (seated, lying down or standing) rests the muscles of the body, but on condition that it goes together with interior restfulness or calm. If someone is worried, anxious, afraid or otherwise unsettled, his muscles will not be relaxed and so he will not be able to rest physically either.

So, for good physical rest, one must feel rested and relaxed. Relaxation supposes interior calm and facilitates physical relaxation. The relation between the psychological and the physical is two-way. By means, then, of physical relaxation, which needs a certain restfulness, one experiences interior calm. Many relaxation techniques, such as transcendental meditation and yoga, are based on this.

Rest can be explained as a "process", an activity that develops with time, by stages:

- The first step is the voluntary decision to rest;
- The second, to stop any activity that makes us tired; physical restfulness consists of this, as it allows muscular or physical relaxation;
- And it must be accompanied by interior or psychological calm.

There are people who have never learned how to rest, or, if they have, don't practice it properly. Others try, but do not go the whole way.

Some people do not manage to rest because they cannot stop and "do nothing"; they are hyperactive, workaholics who prefer not to have to stop and think or remain alone with themselves.

Others stop and take a break, but never relax; they are always on the alert, tense, for one of several reasons:

- Out of fear that something will happen if they lower their guard;
- Because if they relax, they will feel remorse or guilt for wasting their time and not being "usefully occupied";
- For fear that if someone sees them relaxed or "doing nothing" they will think badly of them because they are lazy and with time on their hands.

And so they never attain *interior calm*, which is the stage where one can best rest physically and psychologically.

Sometimes it is not easy to get to the bottom of why someone is unable to practice the three stages of restfulness/stillness-relaxation-calm. But unless he discovers the cause and remedies it, he will find it very hard to rest, at least habitually and not just sporadically in special situations such as annual holidays or week-ends.

To make it easier to rest and fight the effects of chronic stress in which so many people live and work today, the business world dedicated to rest and relaxation has invented and marketed articulated chairs, known as ergonomic chairs, to support the arms, legs and head. *Ergonomics* is the science that adapts products, office equipment, office space and the working environment generally for the efficiency, security and comfort of consumers, users and workers (see Wikipedia for more details).

Ergonomic furniture does in fact help people to feel more restful, but one has to follow through with the process and pass to the stage of relaxation and interior calm, which does not depend on furniture alone but on controlling one's interior world (thoughts, emotions and attitude, memory, imagination and outlook on things), and avoid anything negative that can create psychological tension and cause exhaustion over time.

4.2. Relaxation

When we stop working and start to take it easy, our muscles stop contracting and getting tired, and continue with a certain residual activity called "basal or resting muscle tone". In many people who are anxious, tense, nervous, worried, or hyper-responsible this muscle tone is quite high and with time creates a silent, chronic tiredness, which is not evident in the short term in the form of pain or sensations of tiredness.

To attain a more profound rest of the muscles and the whole body, *relaxation of the basal muscle tone* is necessary, and this varies in depth according to each one's facility to relax. As with everything else in life, one has to learn how to do something well, and this learning process consists of theory and practice. To rest one has to *learn how to relax*. Many people have done so and became enthusiasts of relaxation once they felt its benefits. Others, however, have shown skepticism and even repugnance for anything related to relaxation for years, even their whole lifetime, because they think of it as something that has to do with psychiatry and mental illness, and do not want anyone to think they are mad and, therefore, inferior.

There are different *schools and techniques of relaxation*. Some have acquired much prestige, others less. The best known and popular are yoga and transcendental meditation. In the medical world, the most used is the Heinrich Schultz technique ("autogenic training") and the Jacobson relaxation technique ("progressive relaxation"). In addition, a lot of equipment has come onto the market to help relaxation: CDs with suggestions for relaxing, music, videos, etc. All these can help, but what really matters is that the person wants to learn and practice relaxation skills regularly.

The internet also avails many videos (YouTube), made by professionals explaining how to relax and how to acquire interior calm, the final stage of the rest process and the entrance door to deep rest. So there is no shortage of means for learning how to relax. The problem is in the *determination to practice them regularly*.

We conclude this section with learning how to live without tension and excessive tiredness, so as not to need so much restfulness or relaxation.

4.3. Sleep

We spend one third of our life sleeping. And this is because sleep is a physiological process necessary for physical and psychological well-being. Everyone agrees that to feel well one has to sleep well.

Like most other beings in nature, the human has his rhythms and cycles. The circadian cycle or rhythm of sleep-wakefulness (from Latin *circa*, about, approximately, and *dianus*, "lasting one day") is important for health and happiness. The duration of the parts of the cycle differ from person to person, but they are more alike than different. Therefore, we can say that an adult needs around *eight hours sleep*, and that the best hours for sleeping are at night when there is no sunlight, for this is when the hormone *melatonin* is produced in the pineal gland; this is the chemical substance that acts on the neurons which initiate and maintain sleep. The presence and absence of sunlight, by means of the sight, regulates the production of this hormone in the shape of the Gaussian curve (gradual descent, suppression of production and increase of production according to the cycle of sunlight).

Throughout the eight hours of nighttime sleep, owing to the absence of light, the melatonin production is maximum. To maintain a good quality of nighttime sleep it is important to *keep up the constant rhythm of sleep-wakefulness.*

In other words, one should go to bed and wake up at the same time every day. Changes in this timetable need some days to readjust. If the changes are very frequent, the cycle can be disturbed resulting in insomnia.

The quality and amount of sleep are closely related to physical health and especially to psychological health. It is a two-way relationship; that is, when one is physically ill, one's sleep pattern is disturbed. The opposite also happens: when one does not habitually sleep well, certain physical changes may appear, and more so certain psychological changes. Therefore, taking care of our nighttime rest is a wonderful way of maintaining a good balance between tiredness and rest, and preventing health problems.

To be able to sleep one must pass through several stages. The first is physical restfulness: for example, it is not easy to sleep standing, although some people with serious insomnia manage to sleep anywhere (standing, driving, eating, even speaking). After physical restfulness comes relaxation; then, sleepiness, and the first phase of sleep. Hence, we can conclude that it is not easy to fall asleep unless one is relaxed.

4.3.1 *Sleep and psychological problems*

Sleep is the *best method of physical and psychological rest*, because of the deep relaxation experienced, and its duration of several hours, although this varies from person to person. So when someone does not sleep well for a long time, he will end up physically and psychologically exhausted, easily leading to a state of depression.

In my experience, most of the people who do not sleep well or long enough end up having psychological problems. Therefore, I am convinced that everyone needs to sleep seven or eight hours every day. Those who do not sleep well are expending energy which they do not recover sufficiently. With time, especially after the age of forty, they will have to pay back in terms of psychosomatic illnesses (as already mentioned) and depression.

Many people who accumulate psychological tension or anxiety during the day need a lot of time, sometimes hours, to relax body and mind and fall asleep, and suffer what is called *sleep-maintenance insomnia.* They usually sleep superficially owing to the exhaustion produced by being the whole day in tension; once they have slept the first hours of the night, they wake up often (broken sleep), and can wake up several hours before they should.

When someone complains that he does not sleep, he means he has not slept well. We all have lots of experience in sleeping, which goes back to when we were born. We know from very young what it means to sleep well and to sleep badly. Since sound sleep is very important, we must pay attention to people who complain time and again that they do not sleep well, and refer them to a specialist to find out why and apply a remedy, before the onset of the physical and psychological consequences of chronic insomnia.

Despite everything, sometimes it is difficult to solve the problem of insomnia and we must try out hypnotic medication, as a palliative, not as a cure, for a period of time.

4.3.2 *Measures of sleep hygiene*

Because of the importance of sleep for proper rest, all books on this topic have suggestions for sleeping well. These are the so-called *norms of sleep hygiene.* They work well with people who suffer slight sleep alterations, but not in severe cases which need medication and psychotherapy.

	Measures of sleep hygiene
1	Wake up and go to bed at the same time every day
2	Stay in bed no longer than the time needed for sleep (7:5 to 8 hours)
3	Do not consume substances that excite or stimulate the central nervous system just before going to bed
4	Avoid siestas or long naps during the day
5	Do physical exercise to relax you, but not in the late hours of the day, since it can excite the system
6	Avoid activities that can excite or stimulate before going to bed
7	Take a bath with water at body temperature before going to sleep as it has a relaxing effect
8	Eat at regular hours and avoid heavy meals around bed-time
9	Practice some relaxation technique for 15-20 minutes before going to bed
10	Make sure your bedroom has the right ambience: temperature, noise level, light, bed not too soft nor too hard, etc.

Next I shall elaborate on some of these measures of sleep hygiene.

(a) First, one must avoid consuming certain substances, which are *very available nowadays and which act on the normal brain operations*: tobacco, coffee, drinks containing caffeine (like Coca-Cola and Red Bull), stimulants like amphetamines and cocaine, alcohol, medicines against flu, which contain adrenergic substances that activate the brain, and anti-histamines—which cause daytime sleepiness–, tranquillizers and anti-depressants. Bear in mind that most of these substances can reduce the amount of sleep by producing sleep-maintenance insomnia, or causing superficial, broken sleep that suppresses the REM phase (when sleep is at its deepest).

Tranquillizers and anti-depressants are very useful to induce sleep when the cause of insomnia is a psychological illness. The use of these medicines should be determined by a specialist who will decide the dose, the course of treatment and its duration, so as not to cause an iatrogenic sleep disorder. A good number of patients will need to take this type of medication continually. The same happens with many elderly people with sleep problems. They can clearly benefit from taking sleeping tablets to sleep, provided that one keeps a close eye on their effectiveness and the side-effects over a period of time.

(b) Something else I want to emphasize is the need *to not carry out activities that can excite or stimulate before going to bed*, such as watching very thrilling sports matches, watching movies that arouse the nerves and the emotions (horror and violent movies or those with sexual scenes), having heated discussions, brooding over worries or fears, trying to solve difficult or complex problems, etc. Doing this from time to time means altering one's sleep pattern one night and having to catch up over the next two or three nights. But to do so frequently can make catching up difficult, and so produce insomnia, which prevents one from recovering from the day's tiredness.

(c) Ergonomic *beds, cushions and pillows* have come onto the market and have helped to improve restfulness, night-time relaxation and sleep. These are especially useful for older people who have problems with bones and joints, or chronic sickness connected with breathing, or gastro-esophagus reflux, and who need higher pillows to be able to sleep well.

Another improvement has been the use of *eiderdowns* which facilitate sleep, owing to their light weight; they do not press on the legs or produce a sensation of smothering the sleeper, while keeping the body temperature steady during the cold months. Obviously these are only useful in cold climates. Silent air-conditioners are advisable in warm climates, with a thermostat that keeps the temperature constant, or good ventilation.

(d) Are ear-plugs advisable for noisy places or not? Some experts think they should not be used and one should try to adjust to the ambient noise by getting accustomed to it; this helps raise the threshold of sound tolerance so that one stops hearing the usual noises outside. If one cannot get accustomed, there are some very good brands of ear plugs that can be used to block out noise. In my opinion, the best are those made of foam rubber and are usually available in hotels. Wax and rubber plugs are good for underwater fishing, but not for sleeping because they cause discomfort in the ear-drum and work loose when the head moves during sleep, letting in noise.

(e) If noise comes from someone sleeping in the same bed or the same room because the person snores or moves about a lot, one should take a *polysomnography* to find out the cause, and speak with an ear-nose-throat specialist or lung specialist (pulmonologist) or a neurologist). One of the commonest causes of snoring is the *sleep apnoea syndrome* which, with time, can create serious problems, but which can be properly treated. Agitation during sleep can be due to neurological problems, and some can be treated. It is always useful to look for the cause; what is useless is to just complain. If there is no solution and one cannot get to sleep, it is better to sleep in separate rooms.

(f) When nighttime sleep is insufficient, because it was too short or one slept badly, it is beneficial to sleep a little during the day with a *siesta or by nodding off.* We all know that many people have a siesta because it does them good. Some think it is a waste of time and feel scruples if they take one. The same people cannot help nodding off during the afternoon working hours and take an involuntary siesta with fewer problems of conscience, but which is not so effective because the sleep is more superficial than if one took a proper siesta. Others struggle bravely to not fall asleep in the afternoon and spend more time in a sleepy state instead of having a proper siesta. 20 to 30 minutes are enough for a siesta, whereas those trying bravely to stay awake will spend 60 to 90 minutes fighting against sleepiness; and in some cases, *e.g.* driving vehicles or operating certain machines, etc. it can be very dangerous.

I remember my surprise, as a student, when I heard of a well-known lecturer in neurology who, when he felt sleep coming on, nodded off for a few minutes. He realized that thanks to this his output was much better. This story of an expert in the nervous system gave me the confidence to defend the siesta and short naps when, for whatever reason, one did not manage to sleep enough at night, without altering one's normal sleep pattern, which is to sleep and rest at night and be awake and work during the day.

Another lecturer told me once that there is an old custom known as the "coffee spoon siesta", which some people years ago used to take after lunch and coffee. They held the spoon in the hand and when they fell asleep the spoon would fall to the ground and the resultant noise would wake them up. They were already refreshed and ready to start the afternoon's work. Such siestas last just a few minutes, just long enough to relax the muscles of the hand holding the spoon.

(g) Some people, to avoid the siesta and feeling sleepy after a meal, take drinks containing caffeine (coffee, Coca-Cola, Red-Bull) to keep them awake and alert throughout the day. Since tolerance to coffee is quite fast, they run the risk of becoming addicted and, paradoxically, unable to sleep at night unless they take these drinks, because they suffer the nighttime syndrome of withdrawal.

(h) I would like to insist that our brain has a special need of sleep, which varies with age, but always between 7 and 8 hours. When someone is short of sleep he feels sleepy during the day. It is then advisable to take a short siesta, no more than 30 minutes, so as to not wake up irritable and out of sorts. If the siesta lasts longer, it may be difficult to fall asleep at night, which creates a vicious cycle: take a long siesta, sleep less at night, take a longer siesta, etc.

(i) When someone cannot sleep well at night because of problems of health or work, or because small children keep him or her awake, they must take advantage of the chances they have during day-time to nod off, and this can help make up for lost sleep. To take a nap or two without feeling ashamed or guilty one can make use of long or short trips, or time spent in waiting-rooms, or breaks in work.

Always bear in mind that people who do not sleep the time they need disturb the activity-restfulness, tiredness-rest, tension-relaxation equilibrium. Over time, this produces physical and psychological problems related to chronic tiredness.

(j) Here we need to speak briefly about *sleeping tablets.* These medicines are widely used everywhere, since sleeping problems are very common and methods of sleep hygiene are not very effective. Although the sleep they produce is not as good as natural sleep, it is sufficiently restorative.

The early kinds of *sleeping-tablets* (barbiturates) brought about serious problems of addiction and tolerance (in cases of overdose they were dangerous); new sleeping tablets are ever more safe, whether taken for a short time or for many years. In addition, the latest ones on the market produce high-quality sleep.

There are also several natural products, prepared with plant extracts (valerian, lime, passion flower), which have a sedative effect and can induce sleep in cases of insomnia caused by mild anxiety. What does not work are gadgets manufactured for sleeping, and sometimes available in shops, which produce ultrasounds, micro-waves, vibrations, oxygenated air, etc.

Some people, because of their way of being (anxious, worried, over-responsible, perfectionist) will always find it hard to relax. They will suffer insomnia habitually and will need to take sleeping pills their whole life. Anyone who finds this alarming should realize that there are people who take certain substances almost their whole life (tobacco, alcohol, caffeine, painkillers, medicines for blood pressure, diabetes, etc), and no-one is surprised. No doubt, the best solution is to change the way one is, but very often, from the age of 35-40 years on, this can be very difficult and in fact most people do not manage. It is common for important people and those with heavy responsibilities to take tablets for years without their professional performance and quality of life being affected. Thanks to sleeping pills they can continue to carry out their responsibilities properly.

(k) Lastly, one should realize that *sleep and wakefulness are closely related*: good sleep means a good day ahead, at least physically and psychologically. The quality of the day determines the quality of night-time sleep. A bad day because of problems, worries, contradictions, fears, annoyances and frustrations leads to a bad night, both because one finds it hard to fall asleep and because one sleeps badly, due to tension, bad dreams or nightmares.

If this lasts many days in a row, it can produce insomnia, day-time tiredness and emotional upsets such as irritability, hyper-sensitivity, anxiety and even depression. Hence, the importance of a peaceful life, with no hurry, annoyances, strains, pessimism, worries or fears.

This is attained not by going to a desert island or putting oneself in a magic bubble away from life's problems. It is achieved by being optimistic, having a good sense of humour (which nothing can upset) and being able to cope with frustration (patience).

The important thing is not for the world to be as we would like, so that it does not affect us negatively, but that we become masters of our own interior world, so that nothing or anyone can ever rob us of our peace and joy ("every cloud has a silver lining"). It is as if we were to be vaccinated psychologically against the negative aspects of the world around us. People who do not achieve this emotional independence live in a state of tension and fear, which gives them further tiredness, prevents them sleeping well and cancels the beneficial effects of a good night's sleep.

5 PSYCHOLOGICAL TIREDNESS

Tiredness has different sources, in function of the activity of our human faculties, physical, psychological and spiritual. This distinction can help us understand better the source and the solution of tiredness, because all tiredness, regardless of its source, affects the whole of the person. Therefore, physical tiredness has psychological manifestations, and psychological tiredness causes physical tiredness. Again, distinguishing the kinds of tiredness is very useful for finding a solution based on its source ("dead dog, no more rabies").

Pathological kinds of tiredness that affect the whole person and have their source in psychological tiredness have been known from ancient times. Throughout the history of psychiatry they have had different names: "surmenage" or over-exertion, neurasthenia, psychasthenia. In recent years, these processes of pathological tiredness have come to be referred to as chronic asthenia syndrome and burn-out. These kinds of *asthenia*—which is the medical term used for physical tiredness- have asthenia as the dominant *symptom*; but being *syndromes* (collections of symptoms), they have other symptoms which include those of psychological tiredness: difficulty in concentration, irritability and emotional hypersensitivity, lack of intellectual energy, emotional repugnance for duties and responsibilities.

The *cause* of these kinds of tiredness is prolonged, intense work without sufficient or proportionate time for rest. Constant, prolonged work wastes away physical and psychological energy, which brings about—as I have already said—exhaustion of chemicals in the body and the brain that produce energy.

In the rest of the book I will maintain this separation between the physical and psychological aspects, and make a distinction or separation of the factors that can cause psychological tiredness. I have selected a few of these factors, the ones I think most important because they are more common and affect a lot of people. This list, which is by no means complete, is general enough to include other more specific sub-factors of tension and tiredness. They do not follow any order of importance. Where there is repetition and overlapping is because some factors have aspects in common.

5.1. Preoccupations or Worries

These are defined as "states of disquiet and fear produced by a problematic situation". They have, therefore, a negative connotation: they have a positive opposite "occupations". All of us have preoccupations from time to time, but for some people this is a habitual feature of their life.

To be preoccupied is a vital attitude, and, as with every vital attitude, there are three different aspects or elements:

- The *affective* or emotional element: the fear of something going wrong and making one suffer, and a feeling of tension, impatience, expectation or alert;
- The *cognitive* element: Repeated negative ideas about something that is making one worry. The importance of this element lies in its emotional repercussions ("I shall suffer if it doesn't turn out as I hope", or, on the contrary, "I shall be overjoyed if it works out well");
- The *behavioral* element: the behavior needed to solve the problem at hand.

If the worries are very intense they can *provoke precisely what one is afraid of*, because one does not act prudently or sensibly, but emotionally (fear of failing, making a mess or getting into worse trouble).

Worries create great psychological tension. If they last for a long time, or are intense over a short period of time, one's energy reserves can reach exhaustion point. Obviously people get most worried over matters that cause suffering if they do not turn out well and as one wishes: things one is attached to, such as one's own health or that of family members, one's success or that of people dear to us, in important areas of their lives, such as their material well-being, etc.

These people should be reminded, so as not to worry themselves uselessly, that *no-one can control the external world* and make it according to his liking; but one can *control one's interior world*. By persevering in training oneself psychologically, one learns to be in control of one's interior faculties: thoughts, emotions and attitudes, imagination, memory and one's perception of people and events. In this way one can think, feel, imagine, remember and perceive what one wants to and not what external stimuli dictate. With this interior control, one comes to the point of not becoming "preoccupied" with things, but only "occupied" with them.

In order to not "become preoccupied" or worried, and to stop being a worrisome person, and not end up exhausted, one has to aim more at control of one's interior world than the external world: to wish to have more peace and interior joy than avoid suffering from the problems and failures of the external world.

There are people who think that the world has to be just as they wish it: ideal, perfect, good so that they will not have to suffer, but rather live in a kind of paradise. They refuse to accept that the world is as it is, that there have always been good people and bad, sickness, violence, poverty, injustice and problems to make us suffer. If we "accept" the suffering, we shall stop being afraid of it and suffer much less and not worry so much. *To accept does not mean to get used to it.* To accept is not to complain or moan, not get upset and sad interiorly when one suffers. To get used to something, on the other hand, is to remain passive and do nothing to improve the situation. Therefore, one has to combine acceptance with not getting used to something. Acceptance not only makes it easier to accept unavoidable suffering; it also allows one to find a solution for suffering that is avoidable.

People who do not manage to control their interior world not only suffer an intense negative effect from the world outside, because of their worries and fears, but, because they are affected by its bad example, they can also develop an interior world that is not compatible with their moral or ethical principles. In other words, they think, feel, imagine, remember and perceive, and later behave, against their moral convictions. This morally conflictive interior life gives them continual cause for worry; they worry that they are not doing what they should, together with a constant state of unease, tension, anxiety, dissatisfaction and unhappiness, which results in an increase in tiredness. *Such tiredness is of a moral or spiritual origin*, because it is due to not having a habitual peaceful conscience.

Until one attains sufficient interior self-control, one should "get rid of one's worries" by occupying oneself with other things, sharing one's worries with other people, laughing at one's worries, and so on. All of us have activities that expel worries from our minds for some time. Obviously we should avoid those that make us feel worse afterwards, as happens, for example, with getting drunk, compulsive spending, drugs, pornography, getting into trouble and blaming everything around us (like the tantrums of a small child).

For many people, the brooms that sweep away worries are: watching or playing sports, indoor games, reading, music, films. Afterwards, perhaps they go back to their worries, but differently, because they have rested from them. And sometimes the fact of distancing oneself from worries for an interval of distraction helps them not worry so much as before.

5.2. Routine and daily living

Just as some background music (the kind found in waiting-rooms) helps some people relax, the *habitual stimuli* of every day can cause others to experience tiredness, boredom and satiety which like every situation of tiredness, in this case psychological, goes together with other negative emotions, such as irritability, hypersensitivity, dissatisfaction, sadness and frustration.

Some people, because of the way they are—insecure, stiff, fearful and needing to be fully in control of everything around them—feel more at ease in the same, unchanging, familiar environments, since they have little flexibility to adapt to the changes required by work and extra tension. But even those people who love routine and hate change can after some time begin to feel tired and fed up with the same routine. This happens first and more intensely with those who have more life and energy, the more emotional, who need frequent and varying stimuli to avoid feeling bored and satiated.

This is especially the case of women, who are more emotional than men. Perhaps this explains why they need to change their dress and appearance every day so as to feel different. They also need to add fresh little details of decoration to their room or their house. It is quite striking the amount of objects some women collect in their houses to change their environment and avoid monotony.

We all need to *change our routines* from time to time, to a greater or lesser extent: environmental routines (room, office, house, or car), our usual movements (finding new routes to go from one place to another), ways of dressing, type of ballpoint pens, physical appearance (haircut, accessories, watch, rings) and even the newspaper we read.

We must make some of these changes more or less frequently according to the tiredness caused by the activity in that familiar environment. When the activity is very tiring the stimuli of the environment where we are doing it are loaded with recollections of the tension we experienced there, and the mere fact of seeing that environment reproduces tension and tiredness, *as a kind of conditioned reflex*. It is quite similar to what happens with the fear caused by motor-cars after being involved in accident, or the nausea felt by someone who has received chemotherapy whenever he passes by a hospital.

Often someone who is tired is advised to "have a change of scenery", to go for an outing or to the beach. The advice is intended to help him take a break, for a time, from the work that makes him tired, but also to break off from the *habitual stimuli* that remind him of the activity that has caused the tiredness, and which has produced the tiredness as if by conditioned reflex.

In this sense, it is common for certain kinds of manual workers whose work is boring and repetitive, such as house painters, draughtsmen, carpenters, lorry-drivers, bricklayers, etc. to turn on the radio or listen to music, which are ambient stimuli that give some variety and help them relax, in order to reduce the tiredness produced by routine.

It is worth bearing in mind the negative "subliminal" (subconscious) effect of the habitual, of routine, so as to introduce changes in the environment, in one's way of doing things, such as dressing, eating, walking, etc., and so prevent negative consequences.

I once heard a joke of a bricklayer who always carried cheese sandwiches in his packed lunch, because he liked cheese. One day he started to complain that he was tired of cheese sandwiches. His work-mates suggested he tell his wife to prepare something different, but he said that he was the one who prepared his lunch. A little bit of imagination and creativity are needed to make daily life more pleasant, and not fall into repetition out of the laziness of not having to think how to make small changes to one's life style.

To show why it is good to make small changes and add something new to one's daily routine, I usually give the example of the vegetable salad. If every day we only took lettuce on its own, we would soon get tired of it, but if we add tomatoes, avocado, onion, cucumber, tuna fish, gherkin, oil, salt, vinegar, etc., we do not get tired. In the same way, it is recommended to "embellish" and "garnish" each new day to make it pleasant and less tiring.

5.3. Tension and stress

From the time we wake up and start our daily round, we have to make efforts, acts of the will which use up our energy, make us more or less tense and make us tired. Some days the things we have to do are easy because we know how to do them; other days they are harder, either because we do not know how to do them or they are important because we must do them especially well. This kind require more effort and more attention, and makes us more tense and anxious since we are not sure how they will turn out.

In our lives we have some *days or seasons of greater stress*. Stress is not dangerous, provided it is kept within limits that do not produce pathological symptoms (physical or psychological), as well as a healthy balance between times of stress and relaxation. For some people (the placid, stable, optimistic types) stress control and maintaining the balance is relatively easy. For others, (the insecure, pessimistic, worrying types), it is almost impossible, and they need professional help.

Special care must be taken in situations of very intense *acute stress* (death of loved ones, being laid off work, grave illness, physical or psychological abuse, etc); but sometimes *chronic stress* (less intense but more prolonged) is more dangerous.

- The person who suffers acute stress and the people around him easily notice, and can take the necessary measures and seek help to tackle it and avoid the consequences;
- But the one who suffers chronic stress gets used to living with it and it seems quite normal to him. The people around him do not realize

how serious the situation is and do not come to his aid as in the case of acute stress.

In the case of chronic stress, the sufferer develops the habits of a stressed out life that sink their roots deeper, and are difficult to root out when the pathological effects start to appear. He cannot live without stress, which is like a drug, because it keeps urging him on to give more; he becomes its accomplice, he needs it and accepts it. Over time, and as he gets older, and with less resistance to the psychological tension, the stress starts to produce pathological symptoms, which are not easy to cure since it is difficult to eradicate the cause, namely his deeply-rooted stressful life.

In recent years *relaxation techniques* have spread and multiplied, to fight this ever more common illness of our society: stress. Their life style and heavy workload cause many people to accumulate psychological tension or anxiety. *Stress and anxiety are identical emotional conditions.* But we speak of stress when anxiety is caused mainly by environmental factors, but when the source is in the person himself, for reasons of insecurity or fear, it is called plain anxiety. So we shall speak indiscriminately of stress, anxiety and nervousness or nerves.

Anxiety is accompanied by physical and psychological signs. The psychological ones are sensations of haste, acceleration, worry, restlessness and tension. The physical ones are produced by the activation of the sympathetic vegetative nervous system, which acts on the body by discharging adrenaline.

The sympathetic system tries to prepare the organism for "fight or flight": it is how the body reacts when it detects danger for the physical wholeness/integrity, or the psychological wholeness (self-esteem). When the person is in danger or very afraid anxiety is transformed into *anguish*, which is different from anxiety because it paralyzes and freezes him and renders him helpless physically and psychologically, causing him to succumb to the very danger that gives rise to the fear.

When these emotions (anxiety, stress, nervousness, anguish) are short-lived they do not exhaust all one's energy reserves as these can be restored easily with relaxation. But when they are chronic, that is habitual, they end up exhausting the person and producing the already mentioned psychosomatic and psychiatric illnesses related to stress. Hence, the importance of avoiding chronic stress, and if it cannot be avoided fighting it with an antidote, such as activities and behavior that help the person relax, which we shall deal with in the second part of this book.

5.3.1 *Psychological manifestations of chronic stress*

As stress (or reactive anxiety) supposes a state of sustained psychological hyper-function (state of alert and watchfulness), its psycho-pathological manifestations are a consequence of exhaustion (or depression) of the psychological functions, especially the higher functions (intelligence and will). These symptoms appear in people who suffer it:

- Difficulty in concentrating and remembering
- Slow reasoning
- Finding it hard to take decisions (frequent doubts)
- Loss of interest
- Reduced intellectual stamina (avoid thinking and looking for continuous audio-visual stimuli)
- Obsessions (ideas, images or memories that suffocate and cannot be expelled from the mind)
- Psychological asthenia
- Inconstancy
- Refusing responsibilities

At the same time as the cognitive functions (intellect and will) are diminished, the functions under their control cry for attention, such as the imagination, the psycho-motor functions, the affectivity, one's natural tendencies and sensibility. And these symptoms appear:

- Irritability and anger
- Hyper-sensitivity and mood swings
- Dissatisfaction and sadness
- Impulsiveness
- Psycho-motor agitation
- Interior restlessness
- Impatience
- Confusion
- Sensitive disturbances (intolerance of noise, bright lights, heat and cold, pressure of certain clothing textiles)

The final outcome of a chronic state of stress is usually *depression.* Stress can then be considered as a pre-depressive condition or depression in the making.

5.3.2 *Physical manifestation of chronic stress*

During stress (or reactive anxiety) there is a physiological hyper-function of the sympathetic branch of the autonomic nervous system. If this lasts too long the organs can get damaged with the appearance of the so-called psycho-somatic illnesses:

- Migraine
- Insomnia
- Gastritis and gastric ulcers
- Spastic colitis
- Loss of hair
- Eczema
- Irregular heart-beat
- High blood pressure
- Physical asthenia
- Infections (especially viral)
- And many others that appear in manuals of psycho-somatic medicine.

Stress, besides, is behind other physical alterations such as certain cases of obesity, alcohol, tobacco and other substance abuse because of the anxiolytic effect of ingesting certain foodstuffs, especially sweets, or the energizing effect of certain substances ingested, like coffee and Coca-Cola, which counteract the physical wear and tear of stress.

5.4. Responsibilities

One of the things that is most psychologically tiring is holding responsibilities. Responsibility is defined in the dictionary as "a duty to deal with or take care of something or somebody so that you may be blamed if something goes wrong" (Oxford Advanced Learners). There is a feeling of duty with respect to performing a task which, if it does not work out for those concerned, can produce feelings of guilt, frustration, sadness and anguish.

Responsibility is a positive, beneficial characteristic of one's personality. It means *knowing* what is good for each one and for those around us, and *wanting* to do what one knows is good and avoid what is evil. To do the known and wished for good makes someone happy and feel good, because that is what we are made for. The problem, however, is *being excessively responsible.*

The overly responsible person is one who does good without complete freedom, afraid of suffering if he does not achieve the desired result; or someone who feels responsible for things that are not his to feel responsible for. Some people think the world will come to a standstill if they stop doing everything they are doing (as if they carried the world on their shoulders). Others do not know themselves well or what talents they have, but think they have to do as those who have ten talents. "They bite off more than they can chew". They think they can do everything and must take a leading role in all they do. Instead, they have to learn how to be helped by others how to be more down to earth and realistic, and not build castles in the air. There are many Don Quixotes around who do not want to listen to the sensible advice of the Sancho Panza who try to open their eyes to reality.[1]

To continue with the psychological consequences of being overly responsible. A person who feels responsible for something will notice a psychological tension during the time the responsibility lasts. This tenseness wastes away his psychological energies, producing a sensation of tiredness.

Everyone has responsibilities, but not everyone demands of himself to the same extent. Some have that kind of personality: they tax themselves, are perfectionist, driven by sheer will-power, heightened sense of duty and an excessive sense of responsibility, and expect to carry out their responsibilities to perfection, on time and to everyone's taste. The fear of feeling bad at failing and their strong sense of duty create in them a high level of tension while they are doing the task entrusted to them. And when they fail to fulfil their responsibilities to their liking they experience powerful *feelings of guilt and frustration.*

Because such people are that way and do everything very well, other people tend to load other responsibilities onto them, knowing they will do the job well and on time. Then the person finds himself *continually hemmed in by many responsibilities*, which increases the tension and brings about psychological wear and tear. He cannot say "No" to the requests of others; he thinks it would be a lack of responsibility and of good manners. And since he never says "No", *because he doesn't know how to*, the others think he never says "No" *because he is able to cope*, they load onto him ever more jobs and responsibilities. This creates a vicious circle which, unless broken in time, can end up in psychological exhaustion and mental illness.

Obviously, this is an extreme case, of someone who suffers a serious personality problem (called *anankastic personality disorder).*

Most people are more or less responsible and it can happen that at certain times of their life they are given particularly heavy and important responsibilities, such as a work promotion, the birth of children, looking after sick relatives, difficult financial situation etc., which can make them exhausted. Perhaps they did not know how to ask for help from people around them, and it is necessary to learn how to do this every day.

We all have to *learn little by little to ask for help*, and also to say "No", or "Enough, no more", to "switch off" and rest in situations of heavy responsibility. We must never forget that our first responsibility is to make good use of our own strengths and avoid an illness that makes us unfit to take on new responsibilities.

There are many people who wait for the holidays to give up their responsibilities and rest as much as they can. Holidays are meant for this. But some people, because of their duties, cannot take holidays, such as mothers

---

[1] Translator's foot note: This is a reference to the main characters in the Spanish classic novel, Don Quixote de la Mancha by Miguel Cervantes.

of large families, small shop owners, people who look after invalids etc., and they have to learn how to rest throughout the year. It is easy to rest on holiday. It is not so easy *when one has responsibilities to take care of.* One has to learn how to "disconnect"; in other words, for the time being to stop thinking and remembering things at work, to control one's imagination and stop feeling responsible for the jobs at hand.

This "disconnecting" can be at a superficial level, such as not talking about work and amusing oneself with something completely different. But it can also be at a deeper level, which supposes a change of mentality:

- Not feel the sole responsible for a job (share the responsibility and delegate);
- Accept failure with a sense of humour (this can take away more than 50% of the weight of the responsibility);
- Not make the worth or personal prestige of the work done depend only on its being done perfectly;
- Detach oneself emotionally from the opinions of others when they judge how we carry out our work.

"Sticks and stones may break my bones, but words will never hurt me". Excessively responsible people need to hear that their most important responsibility is for their interior world: *to never lose peace and joy.* And that if they want to be very responsible, they should start by *taking over responsibility more for their interior life* than external tasks. They must give more importance to the things that only they can see, such as peace and interior joy, than to the things other people can see.

For such people their inversion of values (first the external world, then their interior one) is usually due to *their need for the esteem of other people* so as not to feel inferior, useless or a failure. They forget that their fear of failing in their responsibilities and losing the esteem of others results in their losing peace and joy and failing in their interior life. In many cases, too, they end up failing in the external world since their negative emotions prevent them carrying out their tasks and responsibilities properly.

In short, those people who have important responsibilities or are overly responsible (even though their tasks are not very important), get very tense in their ordinary lives. They have *greater need of rest,* and have to learn *how to rest,* and to rest regularly. For example, they can rest by:

- Playing sport or indoor games;
- "Disconnecting" by making a trip (although the longer the trip the greater the psychological tiredness);
- Frequently changing their responsibilities and so resting from the previous one;

- Looking on the bright side—laughter goes with a festive sense of life and so helps one not take responsibilities too seriously;
- Asking for help and advice;
- Delegating some responsibilities;
- Trusting in the sense of responsibility of other people—which means "letting go";
- Putting order into one's sense of responsibility: giving more importance to the responsibility of being happy than of being perfect and successful;
- Not trying to show how good one is at fulfilling one's tasks perfectly, since one can still be serious and responsible and fail occasionally;
- Learning how to say "No"—without feeling bad about it—to new responsibilities before one has finished the present ones, so as not to break the balance between tension and relaxation. Too many responsibilities does not give enough time for rest.

Here are some suggestions to avoid the negative effect of too many responsibilities:

(a) First, one should make a definite effort to rid oneself of the fear of failure, of making mistakes and doing things less than perfectly. If we do not give unnecessary importance to the outcome, we shall concentrate better on the job. *What matters is to do a good job, and not a perfect job.* The good quality of the work done depends on us, whereas the result depends on the people working with us and other unforeseen circumstances. If we think like this, we shall reduce tension considerably. This becomes possible when we do not get upset with the little daily mistakes, disappointments and limitations. "Not getting upset" means not getting annoyed or gloomy, complaining openly or to ourselves when we make a mistake. What really matters is to *try to enjoy doing what we have to do,* and not become obsessed with how it will turn out. If we enjoy doing it we will not get so tired.

(b) Our responsibilities are less likely to stress us if we have *a good scale of values*: know what is really important, what is less important and what is not important at all. Some people think everything is important and that they must do everything very well. As our strengths are limited and more so as we get older, we have to know how to invest what strength we have in what really matters, reach where we can without overtaxing ourselves if we do not want to end up exhausted. If we manage to do what is important we feel at ease and sure of ourselves, although we may not reach the less important things. It is like the ballast of a boat that makes it steady in rough weather.

(c) Sometimes we get the *wrong perspective of things*. It is as if our nose were stuck to the wall and we thought the wall was the whole world; in other words, we think that what we have on hand now is of utmost importance to our present and future happiness. This overwhelms us completely, but it should not. It is times like these that we should listen to the opinions and advice of other people; as they do not have their nose stuck to the wall, they see things as they are and can help us to do so too. The saying goes that "no-one is a good judge in his own case". We can never judge how competent we are and how important things are for the present and future, and so we need the assistance and guidance of an experienced judge.

(d) In my opinion a stable, sure and fixed scale of values can help prevent activism and our becoming overly responsible. I suggest an order of values that can be useful for everyone:

- Our principles and beliefs
- Happy family life
- Work satisfaction
- Affection for friends and acquaintances
- Hobbies and pastimes

5.5. Giving a good impression

Being loved and appreciated by others is a psychological need. It has a lot to do with wanting to feel useful and worthwhile, and so feel well with ourselves. An important factor in determining what we do and how we do it, when someone else is present, is the desire to please, and give a good impression. The need for love is linked to that of being thought well of because we learn from very young that people take great care of what is thought valuable (even keeping it under lock and key), whereas things of little value are not wanted and are thrown into the waste basket.

At the root of this need to please others and feel loved is *self-esteem*, which gives one a feeling of security and confidence and goes together with peace of mind. Because of the connection between psychological tension and psychological tiredness, we can understand that people who feel sure of themselves are more calm and relaxed, and have less risk of psychological exhaustion.

Feeling worthwhile (self-esteem), having a positive idea of oneself, comes about from the interplay between the appreciation of oneself and the appreciation others have of us. In our childhood years our self-esteem comes mainly from other people, those around us; when we get older it comes from within, the consideration we have of ourselves.

People who develop a *feeling of inferiority* during their childhood feel an excessive psychological need to be appreciated by other people when they get older. How this feeling develops is not easy to explain without knowing their personal history, but generally this is what happens: the child depends on the appreciation of others to develop his self-esteem. If the others regard him positively only *because he does things very well* and not for his *interior qualities* (goodness, his upright intentions, his virtues and talents, etc), the child will come to esteem himself only for his successes in what he does, which is what other people see, and not his interior achievements (what he knows, his self-control, intellectual ability, his capacity for effort, struggle, sacrifice, and virtues acquired, etc.), which he knows about better than anyone else.

Everyone with more or less low self-esteem, owing to the intense need to be appreciated by others, feels strongly that he is being judged on his worth and, automatically and from a deeply-rooted habit, becomes tense, like an actor on his first night or someone being interviewed by a panel trying to give the best possible impression. The tension is still greater if he is in the presence of socially important people, because he will feel really worthwhile if he is appreciated by them rather than people of a lower standing.

In more pathological cases, at the prospect of not being regarded positively, such a person will keep away from other people and shut himself up at home. This is a case of *social phobia* or *avoidant personality disorder*.

Many other people, without reaching this extreme, end up *in utter exhaustion,* caused by the permanent tension of trying to please and impress everyone, and the continual fear of not succeeding. They live in a *vicious circle*. Feeling the need to be loved and appreciated by everyone, they think they have to be with other people to make a good impression and feel good, although they are worn out by the tension in trying to do so. When they are not with people who like them, they feel lonely, not loved, and inferior. Then, these negative feelings drive them to seek the company of people they like— in such a way that it becomes an obsession- but they do it wanting to make a good impression and feel loved. The outcome is that they experience once again the tension of wanting to please at all costs, and the fear of not succeeding. Whenever they are with someone, they try to guess what is expected of them, and do it, so as to "buy or win over" his appreciation. They can never be themselves, relax, act naturally or spontaneously, be transparent or simple, because they think other people will see how they really are, and despise them. One must remember that the root of this need is their low self-esteem, which makes them feel worthless and gives them a negative view of themselves.

No-one has esteemed them for what they really are, but according to the impression they give of themselves from their behavior; for what they "do" and not for what they "are".

These people find rest "being in the limelight", making their public happy, and creating a good impression, when they are alone. But as they do not like themselves for feeling inferior, they do not get much pleasure out of this and so do not rest either because, as mentioned already, what is most restful is to enjoy oneself. They only experience the passing relief of not having "to put on an act" while they are alone.

Therefore, besides the time they have *to spend with themselves* every day (not to be alone but to be with themselves), they have to learn how to amuse themselves, "to stay on their own" to have a good time. And how do they do this? Doing over and over again those things that most people do when alone to amuse themselves: reading, manual skills, individual games, fishing, hunting, Sudoku, crossword puzzles, listening to music, watching movies, going for a walk, etc. Generally, the easier and more straightforward these things are the better. And better still if they are inexpensive and can be done in any weather or place or at any time of life. Having a good time with ourselves, we shall like ourselves; liking ourselves, we come to esteem ourselves more, and so the appreciation of others matters less to us. In this way we shall manage to "be ourselves" with other people—we will not have to give a good impression at any price—and the pathological vicious circle associated with inferiority is broken.

On the other hand, so that people with low self-esteem learn how to stop thinking they have "to give a good impression" and to relax when with other people, they have to convince themselves of *the need for interior freedom if they want to be happy*. For this they must acquire sufficient emotional independence with respect to other people and try to get rid of the idea that they must be appreciated and esteemed by everyone. To achieve this, it is very helpful to practice regularly just being oneself, trying not to behave in order to please, and even, when necessary, allow situations where they annoy, contradict or upset others. This will appear impossible to them because for years they have been doing the opposite but from their experience of feeling bad about themselves when they do not manage to make others happy it becomes relatively easy after some time to actually do this. Suspecting that it is not possible is more psychological than real. Besides, the feeling of liberation and independence they feel when they "pass over" someone can be gratifying and encouraging.

Owing to their intense fear of feeling bad and not liked, people with low self-esteem "*get stuck*" when they are asked to be themselves, to be spontaneous, simple, natural, transparent and relaxed in public. Therefore, they should be told time and again to at least try, and start doing it with people who really like them and who will not shun or humiliate them. Once they experience the wonderful feeling of freedom, and realize they have not lost the esteem or affection of others, *they become convinced that it is worth trying to live like this*, and that they are less tense and worn out than before. This process of change is lengthy; it takes time to eradicate a habit of many years. Despite everything, in a few months they will notice a difference, which will drive them forward.

5.6. Boredom

Boredom is related to routine, but one can get bored not only with routine situations but with novel ones too.

Boredom has not only to do with one's usual activities, but also, and especially, *with one's attitude towards them.* Many mothers do the same things day after day, repetitive, trivial and seemingly unimportant, but they do them because they love their husband and their children, and because they want them to feel happy at home, with the meals well prepared and their clothes washed and pressed. This is the *love with which they carry out the bigger duties and the smaller ones of each day.* And this fills them with joy and peace of mind, which are precisely an antidote against the tiredness of routine and prevent boredom. Many other people do small, routine and monotonous tasks which neither bore them nor wear them out because they do them with enthusiasm, passion and love. Such attitudes fight off psychological and spiritual tiredness, though they can make one physically tired, but this usually passes after a good night's sleep or relaxed reading, watching TV or going for a short walk.

On the other hand, there are people who do almost nothing whereas others are always switching activity, like butterflies fluttering from flower to flower, and who feel tremendously bored because they put neither love nor passion into what they do. Their activity gives them neither satisfaction nor fulfilment.

There are individuals who have such a passive personality that they need other people to do things that entertain them. If such people do not appear in their environment, such passive individuals would not know what to do in order to have a good time and to enjoy. In exchange, there are many people who manage to enjoy whatever they do and have a pile of things they enjoy doing "when they have nothing to do". To have many interests and practice them often helps one to enjoy life enormously and not fall into a boredom that drains one's energies. *It is just as exhausting to do nothing as it is to never enjoy what one does.*

Overly responsible people don't allow themselves to enjoy life because they think it is selfish: "Since there are so many things to do and so many problems in the world, what right do I have to enjoy myself?" They only know how to fulfil their duty and very often it gives them neither pleasure nor enthusiasm; they do so from a strict, cheerless sense of "responsibility". Over time they remain fed up with so much sense of duty, dissatisfied and bored to death. To avoid these negative sensations they try to escape in the wrong direction, that is they work more than ever and take on even more obligations. They exist in a kind of binge of activism, so as to keep their minds busy with what they are doing and not have to think if they are happy with what they are doing or even why they are doing it. The outcome of all this can be a serious depression which is hard to treat because it means a complete change of attitude and way of being.

The *origin of excessive responsibility* lies in the attitude of some parents in educating their children. They want their children to be very responsible, make best use of their time and study hard so they grow up to be important and successful. Therefore, they show their displeasure when their child "wastes time" playing with his friends and enjoying his hobbies. They do not let the child think that games and enjoying oneself are good and healthy or that they are a way of resting from his duties and obligations. They impede the child from seeing that when he is rested and happy, he can perform better when he returns to his work. It is certainly good that parents teach their children to work and be responsible, but also to play and "waste time" in things that relax and amuse them.

Others become excessively responsible because from a very early age they had to take on responsibilities which impeded them from playing, and so they thought that play was for other children, but not for them. Sometimes this cannot be helped but it must be borne in mind so that it is remedied as soon as this period of necessity ends in order to allow such persons practice ludic activities (*e.g.* sports and games) with the end goal of counteracting their heightened sense of responsibility.

In short, a proper balance between "obligations" (responsibilities) and "distractions" (interests, hobbies, amusements) prevents boredom and dreariness that can end up draining vital energies.

5.7. Competitiveness

We live in a world that glorifies *the winner.* From a very early stage it has been drummed into us that we have to be among the first, that if we are at the top we shall be happy. And so the *habit develops of continually comparing ourselves with others*, to see if we are better or worse, if we look better than they do or if we have better things than they have. And this creates permanent tension, a state of watchfulness, to try to outdo the others. This competitive habit is shown in the silliest things, like being the first to go at a traffic light, get into a bus and choose the best seat, be served first in a shop or an office, to win at sport or be a supporter of the winning team, etc.

Competitiveness and wanting to be the best and outdo the others, alongside the fear of losing, produce a state of continual tension, together with the psychological suffering (frustration, humiliation and rage) that causes exhaustion. The competitive person, even when he tries to rest by doing things he likes with others, does not manage to rest completely because his competitive habit pushes him to want to win even in recreational activities, such as sport and indoor games, and instead of enjoying himself he becomes bitter and annoyed.

The need to compete and win is much more rooted in people with *low self-esteem*, or with *a stronger feeling of inferiority*, which makes them feel insecure and anxious. They only feel comfortable when they have people around them who are worse off than them *i.e.* persons of an inferior status in what they consider important, (academic results, elegance, health, education, culture, or wealth, etc.)

Competitive types, worn out with competing night and day (even at night they wear themselves out dreaming about competing or agonizing in dreams where they are defeated and humiliated), need to *forget all about competition.*

They should start by not bothering if others are better or worse, and not looking at them as competitors. It will be hard for them to begin with, because the habit is deeply rooted, but after some months trying to cut off straightaway all value judgments they will find it easier. By not judging others or themselves better or worse, they will no longer feel the urge to compete.

To get rid of the tiredness of competing, it is useful to remind such people—and it may be necessary to repeat it often—that *they have retired from the race of success and triumphs* just as sportsmen retire from competition at some point in their life. Instead of looking for new sporting triumphs they must now be content with enjoying the ones they have achieved already.

For this new non-competitive attitude to take root, they must try often and for a long time to let themselves be beaten, or, at least, not try to win at all costs, especially in the little "skirmishes" of each day. For example:

- Let others pass through a door first, or on the pavement or while driving;
- Give way to others when there is a difference of opinion;
- Relax and not get upset when one's team loses;
- Admit that others have better watches, smart-phones or motor-cars, without getting upset;
- Agree that others tell jokes better or know more about one's favorite sport or some other area of knowledge, without getting annoyed.

As seen in the examples, to cease being competitive, *it is not enough to let oneself be defeated externally; much more important is to accept it interiorly.* One must now compete within oneself instead of against others. As one begins to change his competitive mentality, he begins to relax, gets less tired and enjoys the things he does more, because now he does not do them to win, with the tension this creates, but to feel good doing his duty, or serving and giving pleasure to the people alongside him.

5.8. The need to succeed

We all need successes in life in order to feel worthwhile, affirm ourselves and not give way to insecurity and lack of self-confidence. Therefore some degree of success is psychologically necessary, just as food is to keep us fit and well. *The problem is in the excess.*

In the previous section, I mentioned how exhausting it is to compete to win in everything one does. I now want to say how success is a necessary part of rest, properly understood.

People who feel they must succeed at any price are in the same predicament as perfectionists: *for them the outcome of whatever they do has to be perfect*, lest the uncertainty of the result and the fear of not attaining perfection cast a dark shadow on their performance, and is responsible for their permanent state of tension which, with time, leads to exhaustion.

People who simply need success to be happy live in unrelieved tension since they apply all their energies to everything they are involved in to be sure of succeeding. This need is precisely their weak point. *They depend on success in order to be happy.* Whereas the fear of failing and making a mess and their lingering doubts about whether they are doing well or badly add even more tension. By the end of the day they are overwhelmed and sooner or later reach a point of deeply-rooted, utter exhaustion; their life is no life at all.

A typical case is that of students who *live tormented by the fear of failing.* The fear lifts for a time when they study harder. But too much effort in study to make sure they pass together with fighting the fear of failing leaves them no time for resting and having a good time. And so they upset the balance between tiredness and rest, and the quality of their study is reduced. When they see they are not improving, because the material "doesn't enter" their tired heads, the fear of failing returns. And so they work even harder, grow more tense and worried, get still more tired and less effective; and so there closes the vicious circle which will end up in the failure they are afraid would happen.

There are many examples of how the pressing need to succeed and the fear of failure can *actually bring about failure.* There comes to mind an interesting case. It is that of an engaged couple. Because they love each other so much, they fear failing in their relationship, which leads them to be ever on the watch, checking on the other person so as not to lose him or her. The result is that they "suffocate" one another, and the relationship ends because it did not flow freely.

It is common for people too obsessed with success to become so tense at the prospect of failing that they get stuck and *provoke the failure they fear so much.* When the experience of getting stuck and failing happens several times, it can produce a fear of any kind of appraisal or test, which adds a further complication to their exhausted condition.

Some may think I have described extreme cases that have nothing to do with them, and so they do not feel very bothered. But, although I have sketched a caricature of what happens in pathological cases, many people, if they underestimate the risk of addiction to succeeding, can also fall victim and end up in a state of stress which, sooner or later, will produce symptoms of psychological exhaustion.

5.9. Other people

Any normal person, when he is together with other people, tries not to upset, scandalize, worry, contradict them or make them suffer in any way and if possible to do just the opposite: to be pleasant, make them happy, help, praise and console them when appropriate. This means being constantly alert so as to know what can upset and what can give pleasure in order to do the latter and avoid the former. The whole purpose of this is to not feel bad by making others suffer, but to feel good by helping them feel good. This positive attitude towards other people means a certain tension, which is a bit unpleasant, but which is offset by our feeling good when we realize that, as a result, other people like us and appreciate us.

The people most likely to suffer psychological exhaustion from a sustained and heightened social tension are those who are excessively concerned about others, because they want to please them and not annoy them. Even those people who have a normal concern for others and who spend many hours a day with people, as happens with front desk personnel or those whose work is to deal with lots of people, run this same risk.

Such people must apply an adequate counter-measure, namely, to *rest from other people.* They have to dedicate time to themselves, enjoy being with themselves, relaxed and enjoying themselves. They can do exercise, go for a walk, listen to music, watch a movie, make things with their hands, read or "just do nothing", but quietly and reflectively. It will not be easy for people who are not "friends with themselves" or those who feel guilty when they are "not feeling concerned" for other people. They are very good at caring for others, but poor at taking care of themselves. They have to learn to "take care of the caregiver", that they "cannot give what they do not have", which means spending time charging their batteries if they want to be of use to others. Otherwise, they will end up psychologically exhausted.

As one grows older, *psychological energy and stamina diminish*, just like physical energy. We easily accept the fact that top sportsmen retire while quite young, because their energy is not what it has been. But we find it hard to accept that we no longer have the psychological energy of our youthful years. From the age of forty one's energy starts to decline. To prevent this, one must learn how to "be there less" for the others. How to do this:

- Stop being indispensable;
- "let go" of people so they learn how to cope on their own;
- Stop being available for everyone and at any time;
- Allow younger people to take over family, work and social responsibilities;
- Learn to take a back seat in the lives of the people around us;
- Not want others to count on us, ask our opinion and our permission for everything.

People with a *very strong, deeply-rooted habit of living for others* find it very hard to change; they think they are useless, that they are a failure and life is empty, and they go through a kind of withdrawal syndrome when they are not helping others. This is the case of mothers who have had many children or relatives to look after, and when they reach 40 or 50 the children no longer need them as before or they give more time to friends or are thinking of getting married, etc. Then they feel they have no one to love and be loved by in return, which is usually called the "empty nest syndrome".

Every mother, and every kind of caregiver, should continue to *foster friendships and relationships outside the circle of people they usually care for*, so as to rest from the exhausting effort required by being always at the call of other people, and for the day when they will have no-one to care for. Moreover, in their free time—which are moments to "care for themselves"—they should cultivate interests and activities that help them relax, and continue with them when their social circumstances change. In this way they will avoid the crisis that can occur when the activity that took up so much effort (energy, time and affection) over a long period comes to an end.

5.10 Perfectionism

We have already spoken of the *exhaustion brought about by feeling obliged to do everything well, to perfection, or almost perfectly*. It is exhausting because the unremitting effort to do everything possible for things to turn out properly, well ordered, perfect, correct, just right and cause admiration produces continual tension. And besides, because total perfection is not achievable, a feeling of dissatisfaction, frustration and disappointment remains, which does not allow one to feel happy and at ease with one's performance. Not even with the things around us, because we look at them time and again with a critical eye to discover the imperfections and how to improve them.

Besides, as *perfectionism* is an "obsession"; the one who suffers it not only wants to do things perfectly, but wants others to do so too, because he cannot bear things around him being less than perfect. It is a phobia of the imperfect and disorderly, of ugliness, lack of punctuality, slovenly appearance, and bad manners. Phobias always produce anxiety when the object or situation causing it is present. And since the world is not perfect, the perfectionist finds himself in a permanent state of anguish which wears him out.

The way to treat a phobia is to get accustomed to whatever stimulates it. This is a process called "desensitization": it can be "systematic", when it occurs gradually, or by "implosion" when sudden. In practical terms it means that the perfectionist, worn out by his phobia against any kind of imperfection and his obsession for perfection, should of his own will do something imperfect every day, or should witness imperfect situations and try to remain relaxed and not complain or get upset interiorly. Better still if he makes fun of the disorder, the not keeping time, the shoddy job, since good humour is the best antidote against over-dramatizing.

For such people to accept the desensitization treatment they must first be convinced that to pursue *the path of perfection and the ideal* (to be ideal, to be perfect and to have everything just as it should be) *is condemned to failure*, because it is not achievable. What is easily achievable is "to improve", but not be perfect. It is not easy to be convinced of this. Sometimes one can be, but only when it is too late, once psychological exhaustion has set in, in the form of depression, frustration or disillusionment.

After being convinced to abandon the pursuit of the perfect, one must start to *change in practice*, which can be done once one knows what has to be changed. The best is to make a list, as detailed and complete as possible, of those things that the person tries to do "to perfection" every day. Next, he should start to do badly the smallest and simplest things on the list, which means doing them as he would not like them to be done and without losing his sense of humour or becoming annoyed or downcast. At the same time, he must try to put up, calmly and cheerfully, with the things done badly by people around him.

To stir the imagination of perfectionists and the overly responsible, I suggest a list of things, many of them trivial and silly, that can easily be done badly, and which are "good training" for accepting imperfection in other things that are more important and hard to put up with. For example:

- Get out of the bed on the 'wrong" side;
- Take a shower and get dressed in the wrong order;
- One day leave the bed unmade;
- Sit down at table for breakfast at a different place to the normal one;
- Not order books on the shelves when they have fallen over;
- Leave the TV remote control just anywhere;
- Leave the curtains or shutters half closed or not closed at all;
- Leave the bedspread untidy;
- Do not collect the crockery after a meal;
- Leave the WC lid raised
- Park the car on the yellow line;
- Arrive a few minutes late for an appointment;
- Not straighten a picture on the wall;
- Not straighten the mat or the carpet.

By not doing things as we have convinced ourselves we must do them, we rest from the fatigue caused by routine, monotony and "perfection". We also develop a sense of freedom or liberation in our daily lives. Freedom is always psychologically restful, since it is contrary to coercion, and the oppressiveness of all kinds of rigidity, obsession and addiction.

5.11. Giving

Giving things and giving oneself to others is gratifying because it produces positive emotions, such as contentment, satisfaction and a feeling of wellbeing. These positive emotions cancel out the negative ones that come with tiredness; they also forestall the tiredness of ordinary work. Giving has to do with love. Love pushes one to give. And love is the "best medicine" for being happy, the most powerful and inexhaustible source of energy and, therefore, the *best antidote to tiredness.*

Some people spend their whole lives giving themselves to others (family and friends, works of charity, NGOs). These are charitable, selfless people who want to help whenever they can. It is obvious that it is much healthier to be generous, selfless and charitable than the opposite, selfish, self-centred, vain, miserly and stingy.

However, a problem arises when someone thinks that he is obliged to give on every occasion and to everyone, *which is when he loses the freedom of giving*, and feels guilty when he is not giving more. This "need" to give what he senses the others need (even if they don't need, but he needs to give anyway to feel worthy of being accepted, esteemed or loved), becomes a weight around his neck and produces nervous wear and tear and a feeling of emptiness. In any case, giving does not mean just giving material things, but giving oneself to oneself: that is one's time, one's opinion, one's tastes and one's peace of mind.

It is true, as Scripture says, that "there is more joy in giving than receiving" (Acts 20:35). Therefore we get pleasure from giving. But unless we do so freely, "because we feel like it", rather than out of fear of feeling bad with ourselves (selfish, stingy), giving does not give us joy, but suffering instead. The one who acts from fear is not free, but a slave of his fear. Freedom consists in the power to do good because it is good, and for no other reason, such as "because I was told to", or "because if not I would feel bad". I have said already that without freedom there is no happiness, which is what helps us rest best.

Sometimes when certain people are asked why they give so much, they say they do it because "they want to". What they really mean is that this was so to begin with but after some time giving became a kind of "psychological need", and they no longer do so freely. Consequently they don't experience the joy they expect to, but only the relief of not feeling selfish, guilty or ashamed of themselves.

They need to *get back the true freedom of giving*. To do this they have to stop giving things or themselves to others for a period of time proportionate to the time they spent not giving with a free spirit. They must let others give to them for a long period of time. In other words, they must learn how to receive help, affection, and gifts without feeling obliged to give back more than they receive so as not *to feel indebted.* They have to be told, and to understand, that by letting others give to them, they are already giving something, namely enabling others to live charity.

It is good for them to learn to see others give and give themselves, without feeling they have to emulate them so as not to be considered worse off. They must learn, then, not to compete with others in being good and charitable. "Let every wayfarer follow his own path". The fact of seeing generous, magnanimous, open-handed people does not mean they must do the same *so as not to feel bad or in order to feel better.* We have to give "because we feel like it", with interior freedom of spirit.

5.12 Fear

The sensation of fear and apprehension produces psychological and physical tension, and if it lasts a long time, it ends up exhausting a person. Like everything else in the human being, fear has *its function and its usefulness.* But if it is excessively intense, as in panic attacks, or lasts long, as with phobias or hypochondria, it eventually destroys one's psychological equilibrium and wears away one's psychological stamina.

The element that is common to all possible fears is *suffering.* All fears are fear of suffering, of having a bad time. The real solution for fearful people is to *learn to suffer with good spirits,* to put on a good face. This is what the masters of the ascetical life have always taught: to practice suffering for a good motive, to increase one's facility for suffering and so reach the point of not fearing it anymore. Those who manage this still suffer, but less than those who fear it. The fearful man *suffers through and through.* He suffers before, imagining all possible sufferings; he suffers during; and he suffers afterwards, for fear that the suffering will come back. The fearful, then, are trapped in a prison of suffering because of the very fear of suffering. And such habitual suffering is completely exhausting.

Nowadays, there is an *epidemic of fear of suffering.* It is there in people who over-protect their children and want to prevent them undergoing any kind of suffering, however small it may be. The prevailing mind-set rejects suffering completely.

Everyone agrees that what one does not learn as a child is more costly to learn when one becomes an adult. Children who do not learn to suffer and overcome their fear of suffering *will become fearful when they grow up and will develop different kinds of pathological fears or phobias.* To fight their fears some will resort to alcohol, pain-killers, anti-depressant drugs and tranquillizers; to protect themselves from the fear of illnesses and other dangers they will go to fortune-tellers, who will give them a false sense of security, to vegetarian diets to prevent cancer, homeopathy, medicinal herbs, Omega 3, superstitions, amulets, Power Balance bracelets, etc.

To say that children have to learn to suffer *does not mean bringing back corporal punishment* but letting them learn the hard way and burn their fingers, and peel their own fruit and remove the bones from the fish themselves—to give some simple examples—and learn to stand up for themselves, and not moan when they don't have what other children have; and that they look for what they need or are missing without running to their mother's apron strings or their father's strong arms.

In short, it is good to let children suffer what they have to suffer without allowing them to complain or throw tantrums or at least tell them that this is not the way to behave if they want to grow up tough. Often it is not enough to let them go through a bad time and encourage them to bear the suffering without complaining. They also need to see *the good example of tough parents and educators* who know how to put on a good face whenever they encounter problems, sickness, contradictions and suffering in general. "Example is the best teacher". If you want your child to be hardy, brave and determined, lead the way, set the right example.

5.13 More haste less speed

Doing things *in a hurry*, or having a sensation of *interior hurry*, although one may be doing nothing, produces psychological tension. Living in a hurry leads to progressive and heightened tiredness.

Some people are *greedy for time*. They cannot waste time, as if the minutes were precious golden coins. Doing nothing or having to wait while doing nothing makes them so tense psychologically that they get annoyed and worn out. Either they get worn out with doing too many things too quickly, or with not being able to do things as quickly as they want because other people are stopping them. They tend to get annoyed often because the world is not going along at their pace, and there are obstacles in the way of their going as fast as they want. This permanent state of annoyance and frustration doesn't let them enjoy the nice little things of everyday life, things that could relax them and help them rest. Thus, the balance between tiredness and rest leans on the side of tiredness.

On the other hand, the speed with which these people live is due to the *sensation that they have many things to do*: things which they *oblige themselves* to do. Their greatest joy, and perhaps their only one, is the relief they feel whenever they finish something and feel liberated from it. Besides doing things in a hurry, they tend to do several things at once, which makes them much more tense than someone who does only one thing and does it calmly. Seeing others do things slowly irritates and annoys them, and makes them feel resentful at their slowness, a resentment that makes it still harder for them to enjoy life and to rest. Seeing the incompetence, slowness and inefficiency of other people—according to them—they react by doing the things themselves, cramming even more things into their already over-loaded timetable and of course becoming still more exhausted.

These people remind me of the rabbit in *Alice in Wonderland.* Alice calls out to the rabbit but, instead of stopping to chat, he draws a big watch from his pocket and replies "Oh dear, Oh dear, I shall be late" and disappears running off. The first time this happened I thought the rabbit must be someone important, at least the Administrator of Wonderland. But after reading the whole story I didn't understand what he was, and I came to the conclusion that he was just "over-stressed". Whereas Alice celebrated her "un-birthday" every day of the year, except the day of her birthday, the rabbit spends his whole life "running for run's sake". I usually show my patients the difference between Alice and the rabbit so they can ask themselves which one they are more like. I also encourage them to learn from the fable of the hare and the tortoise. The tortoise wins because he knows how to go at the speed his nature allows. He does not get tired because he makes no attempt to go faster than he can. Besides, we should take note of the wisdom in the phrase attributed to many personalities of history: "Dress me slowly because I am in a hurry".

There is a close *relation between haste and anxiety*, which makes one tense and worn out. The person who does things in a hurry gets tensed up; the one who does them slowly relaxes. Hence most relaxation and rest techniques include dong nothing or doing something slowly (yoga, tai-chi, taking a stroll, listening to music, sitting on the terrace to drink coffee and chat, etc.).

For people under pressure to be able to rest they have to learn a few things:

- Do nothing useful or important from time to time;
- Do what you have to do but slowly;
- Do one thing at a time and do not think of the next until you have finished the first;
- Not tense up when you see that others are different and do not try to do many things or do them quickly. Each person is as he is and goes at his own pace.

When they try to "change gear" they realize their mistake was to do things to feel good instead of *being happy independently of what they are doing.*

People who live fast and get through many things think that this is the way to happiness. On the other hand, those who are more reflective than active prefer to take it easy, enjoy what they are doing instead of rushing to finish it so as to enjoy the temporary relief of getting rid of an obligation. These people get less tired and enjoy themselves more, and rest from what they have done by doing something new.

5.14 Activity

We have already spoken of the link between doing many things and psychological tiredness. Now I shall explain how important it is to *stop one's activity* in order to rest.

From time to time we need to stop and rest, but not just stop externally. We have to *stop interiorly*: that is, to stop thinking about what we have done or how it came out; not think about if others liked it or not, or if they have thought well of us or not when they saw what we did and spoken about it with others. Also we have to stop thinking about what is still to be done, if we shall have time to do it, if we shall do it well, and the consequences if we do not or if we do not do it on time.

Often what can tire us most is to think of what we have done or half-done or what has yet to be done. When we think of this we lose our peace of mind, worry and do not enjoy life.

Some people suffer a *psychological dependence on the world around them, and on the opinion and esteem of the others*. In order to feel good they need others to think well of them. They think that this can only happen if they are responsible and finish everything to the letter, as I have already explained in the section on resting from responsibilities.

Such people have to learn how to be more *reflective*, and enjoy looking at the things that they or other people have done. It can be very restful to put one's head and one's heart in the things one is experiencing or is about to experience. This is especially so in the case of things that are beautiful, good and true, like the harmony of good music, the beauty of a landscape, a work of art, a building, the goodness of people, animals or things around us. This explains why there are people who choose to rest by listening to music, admire works of art in galleries, walk through cities with beautiful buildings, hike in the mountains or walk by the sea, or simply look at children at play with their simplicity and wonderful spontaneity, chat calmly with a good person or someone knowledgeable, see good films and read the classics. These activities are neither "useful" nor "important", but they produce positive emotions which are the antidote of the negative feelings and emotions caused by tiredness.

I take for granted the importance of carrying out well one's duties as people of responsibility and integrity, but I have stressed the need for reflection in order to lead a balanced life and avoid the excesses that lead to exhaustion.

5.15 Helping others

This section complements the one on resting by means of giving because in helping others we give something of ourselves, such as time, energy, knowledge, money, things, etc.

Helping others gives us positive feelings and emotions and can be a way of resting when tired. But if it becomes an *obsession or a mania* that prevents us from helping ourselves to take it easy, enjoy life and reflect, it can be a source of chronic tiredness. It is not easy to help others well, or help them in what matters in life—namely to live each moment of their life with cheerfulness and peace of mind—if we are not able to help ourselves first. "No-one gives what he doesn't have". We must begin with ourselves, otherwise we shall "sell advice to the others and keep none for ourselves", and not practice what we preach. We must be the testing-ground for ourselves first.

The Christian commandment to love one's neighbor as oneself takes for granted that we both know and practice the duty *to love ourselves.* And so it proposes that we love others as we love ourselves. If one loves himself and not other people, he is not living the commandment; but neither is he living it if he loves others but not himself.

On the other hand, to not help ourselves by wearing ourselves out and endangering our physical and psychological health, would be *to displease* God, from whom we have received freely many physical and psychological talents which we must look after and not mistreat.

Some activities cause chronic tiredness, above all mental tiredness, and must be laid bare in an examination of someone who complains of or shows symptoms of tiredness. Once the activity that causes the tiredness has been identified one must find out why the person works to the point of chronic tiredness. Often it is because he has to carry out that activity to *satisfy some need resulting from psychological imbalance.* When the tiredness is treated, besides helping the person rest, it is essential to solve the personality imbalance to prevent relapses. Occasionally the reason why certain activities lead to exhaustion is a family or social situation. In these cases, the problematic situation has to be resolved and if this is not easy, in conscience it must be attempted.

***

Here ends our study of the factors that could cause chronic tiredness unless controlled, or unless some of the activities to assist rest and relaxation are not practiced, which is our next chapter. With the examples given and the corresponding explanations, it is easier to make a diagnosis and find solutions.

6 RESTFUL ACTIVITIES

In the previous section I dealt with activities and attitudes that can lead to intense, chronic tiredness. I focused on the ones which, from my clinical experience, I consider lead most frequently to pathological exhaustion (psychasthenia, neurasthenia, over-exertion, chronic asthenia, burn-out), and which can produce physical and psychological disorders, with suggestions on how to prevent them.

In this section I shall explain the beneficial aspects of certain activities to prevent and treat tiredness, both normal and pathological. There are many other activities that are good for resting, which the reader can add to his personal list. One simple rule to know if an activity is good for resting is if it produces *short-term and long-term positive emotions.*

6.1. Physical exercise

I have given this section the title above, and not "sport", to differentiate it from competitive sport, and I have already pointed out the stressful effects of competitiveness. I do not mean that competitive sport does not help to rest, above all from the psychological point of view, but it is necessary to "know how to lose" in order to avoid the remedy being worse than the sickness. If one gets annoyed and frustrated and too upset at losing it is better to just do physical exercise.

It is also good to distinguish between *sporadic* exercise and *regular* exercise. *Regular* exercise is more beneficial because the body gets accustomed to exercising—it is kept fit—and the person tires physically and rests psychologically without suffering at all. If someone is not fit, he will probably suffer during and after exercise, and this suffering will go together with negative feelings and psychological tension. If exercise is initiated step by step this can be avoided.

The best physical exercise is *aerobic* because it gives the organism time to adjust to the effort, one breaks into a sweat and gets tired without suffering. There are gentle exercises in which one does not sweat, like walking, which are good for losing a few calories and to relax, but they are not intense enough to produce psychological rest, unless one walks for three hours continuously.

From the physical point of view, some exercises are better than others, according to the number of muscles that are involved. The more muscles involved the better. This happens in swimming, tennis, squash, gymnastics, handball and basketball. From the psychological point of view it is important to "break into a sweat" and reach the point of painless tiredness. Better still if done in a natural setting, such as outdoors.

The body-mind connection is well known and widely accepted. Hence the saying "A healthy mind in a healthy body". Exercise produces an *increase in the production and liberation of endorphins* (endogenous opioids), which cause a psychological sensation of well-being and a feeling of elation and energy. On the other hand, the muscles which tense up and tire with the sustained stress, and afterwards produce a feeling of tiredness, are not the ones that get tense during physical exercise. Owing to the equilibrium between the agonistic muscles and the antagonistic muscles, when one does exercise the relaxed agonistic muscles tense up and the tensed antagonistic muscles relax with the stress. This is one of the causes of physical rest produced by exercise. After physical exercise, the whole body relaxes and this lasts for hours accompanied by psychological wellbeing, which neutralizes the negative physical and psychological sensations of stress.

Moreover, during physical exercise, the intense bodily sensations produced attract the attention of the person concerned and *make him forget altogether or distract him from the worries and tasks* that have caused the stress, helping him rest from them while exercising. After exercising the worries may come back, but it will be differently, more detached and less intense, emotionally more remote, making the person less tense. It is similar to what happens when we go to bed with something on our mind and the next morning, after not thinking of it for eight hours, it has grown less important and stressful. This has given rise to the expression: "I must talk to my pillow about it", which is what some people do when they have to make an important decision, so they "sleep on it" and see the solution more clearly the following morning. These are some of the reasons why physical exercise can produce physical and psychological rest.

6.2. Enjoyment of the senses

I have already said that what helps us really rest is to stop doing what makes us tired and do something we enjoy instead. If we enjoy doing our duties we will not need to go out of our way to rest. But as this is not always easy, we shall have to keep some restful activities in reserve. Many people try to rest with *pleasant sensations* produced by stimulating the senses, especially the eyes, such as TV, cinema, photography, Internet.

The senses are the point of entry to our interior world. All sensible perceptions produce changes in our state of mind and these emotional changes trigger off other psychological functions such as memory, imagination and thoughts. Besides, they affect the physical organism positively or negatively, according to the emotion released by the sensations. Good film directors are very aware of our emotional reactions and cleverly use images, sound-track and dialogue to produce the emotions they want and make the film a success. How often we have wept, laughed, been terrified, fallen in love or get excited watching films!

Our ordinary life, especially in big cities, is invaded by loud noises, sensational advertisements, strong smells, extremes of cold and heat. All these create a deep emotional deposit of tension, haste and fear which over time produces tiredness and excess. As an antidote we need contrary sensations, such as beautiful images, pleasant smells, warm temperatures, silence and soothing sounds which help us rest and restore psychological well-being and physical relaxation.

If the perceptions (rational interpretations of physical sensations) are pleasant, it is because they produce pleasant emotions. Some people badly need to perceive pleasant things—they have a thirst for sensations—so as to neutralize the negative and unpleasant emotions and sensations they experience in daily life. These people feel empty, frustrated, dissatisfied, embittered, sad and anxious. Therefore, they eagerly look for pleasant perceptions as a counter-measure to their negative feelings and emotions.

Others also eagerly seek pleasant perceptions, but because they are *addicted* to them, and when they are missing they have withdrawal symptoms. They need to hear music continually that helps them along, to see films or programmes they like, look into the street to see everything that is going on, smoke when they feel like it, eat their favourite food, use their favourite perfume or cologne or be close to the person they love most. One risk of this abuse of the senses is familiarity and getting too used to what they like which causes a *loss of sensitivity* to pleasant stimuli, and which needs ever more intense and stronger stimuli to feel as they did at first. This ends in greater addiction still and in an emotional instability derived from the frequent emotional changes that go with addictions; there is a big emotional difference between having the stimulus and missing it. In every addiction the *balance is always negative* because one spends more time missing the stimulus than enjoying it.

A rational, balanced use of pleasant sense stimuli is best. One should never become satiated, but always be able to look forward to them; in this way, one's sensitivity is maintained and one can enjoy them time and again without becoming addicted.

Moreover, enjoyment of the senses—taste, sight, hearing, smell and touch—must be accompanied by a parallel enjoyment of the *internal psychic functions*—imagination, memory and thought. Techniques of reflection and meditation to deal with stress-related problems are based on these. The use of the external senses makes us depend more on the world outside. On the contrary, the use of the internal senses or functions only makes us depend on the marks left by our experiences of life and elaborated by our cognitive processes. This makes us more independent of the outside world and more autonomous.

Nowadays in Western society excessive importance is given to the external senses in the pursuit of happiness. This explains the rapid growth in cosmetics, audio-visuals, beauty products, music and everything to do with the pleasures of touch. This culture has produced people *hungry for very quick and very intense sensations*, people who cannot bear silence, or boredom, to go hungry, having to wait, reflection and meditation. The search for and continual consumption of intense external sensations gives people "indigestion" and wears them out and renders pleasant sensations useless as a means of rest. To prevent this, I insist once more on the need to maintain a *good balance between sensations and contemplation or meditation.*

6.3. Music

When one goes to the cinema or watches a movie at home, he is aware of the importance of the sound-track to create the emotions the film director wants us to feel. We have also witnessed the hysteria of young people at rock and jazz concerts. When we watch a symphony orchestra or opera on TV and we see the enthusiasm and long applause, we can understand *the power that music has to produce intense positive emotions* (joy, enthusiasm, passion). Therefore, in many places where people have negative feelings, such as a dentist's waiting-room, background music is played to induce positive feelings.

Music, then, can be a good means for relaxation and enjoyment when we feel tired. Sometimes, if one has already reached psychological exhaustion, it can happen that he loses the capacity to experience the pleasure of music or other positive sense stimuli. Therefore, it is good *to use music regularly and before it is too late.* The best music for resting is the kind we like most but, and though I am not an expert, the best for relaxing is opera or classical choral or symphonic music. The human voice is the best musical instrument, and the voices of opera singers or choirs is the most cultivated. Generally, if a good voice is harmonious it produces positive emotions, even when unaccompanied. Mothers know this very well from the soothing, hypnotic effect of lullabies on little children.

Nowadays, many young people, and not so young, listen to music from getting up to going to bed, in order to feel good or be entertained. MP3s, MP4s, IPods and mobile phones allow many people to go along the street, travel and wait with earphones in place listening to their favorite music. As in films, the lives of such people have a soundtrack that evokes the desired emotions. This has its disadvantages, as it can lead to isolation, addiction and not thinking. To think is to dialogue with oneself, which allows us to know ourselves and be friends with ourselves. So much background music means we neither speak nor listen to ourselves. So, I suggest that to relax and rest one should use music in moderation, and avoid turning it into a means for escaping from oneself, as well as an addiction.

6.4. Cinema

Cinema, which is a fairly recent invention, dating back to the end of the 19th century, is a new version of classical theatre which the ancient Greeks used superbly to achieve two ends: to vent negative emotions by projecting them through the characters—a psychological process called *catharsis*–, and evoking positive feelings among the spectators by means of identifying with the character who is triumphant, courageous, virtuous, handsome, etc. We triumph, love and suffer with the protagonist, we live a different life from our real one for an hour or two, and we rest from the problems and burdens of our personal lives. The fact of submerging ourselves totally, head and heart, into a world distinct from the ordinary helps us to distance ourselves from the routine, and to rest. It is like a fresh breeze on a hot summer's day.

One danger of cinema is that it can make it hard for us to *face the difficulties and sufferings of real life.* When we have to return to a situation that makes us suffer and feel stressed after "escaping" in the movie, we can feel repugnance, annoyance and sadness, because we still long for the world of fantasy in which everything turned out well for the principal character. People who spend hours and hours watching films or TV series to escape from reality find it increasingly harder to face up to real life. This escape mechanism can make a person feel guilty for abandoning his duties. Thus, it is important to insist again that this means of relief and rest from stress must be used with moderation, avoiding escapism and addiction.

6.5. Reading

To read profitably one should sit and concentrate on what one is reading. To be seated is restful physically. And to be focused on what one is reading, which is usually entertaining and amusing, helps us stop thinking about what worries or stresses us, and about what usually occupies our minds. While we are reading we rest from our usual worries and occupations. If our worries are very intense, it is advisable to *read things that hold our attention*, for example those which have to do with an interest or topic we are enthusiastic about, such as cars, contact sports, deep sea diving and others related to the ocean, etc; or those with a very exciting plot, like thrillers and suspense stories; or those with very appealing characters, physically or psychologically.

For many people the best books to read are *spy thrillers or murder stories.* Some think these are a waste of time since they are all alike and tell us nothing new; people like this think they have to find something useful in whatever they do. Precisely for this reason they must learn how to "waste time" reading such novels since, despite being insubstantial, they can arouse positive feelings simply because they are interesting. And it will not be a waste of time, since the intellect is not the only thing that counts.

As happens with cinema, it is equally important for the books to produce positive feelings which cancel out the negative feelings and emotions that go with tiredness. Generally, the books that produce positive feelings are those in which the good characters are very good and the bad characters are bad, and where the good ones win, with the book ending well.

When someone has a taste for good literature, he *never feels lonely*, which is a negative feeling, because he grows fond of the characters who are always at his beck and call whenever he needs to call on them. And if the books are good—in the sense given above–, the characters do not make the reader suffer, but give him much joy since they do not deceive or disappoint, but win out in the end. Good reading is a worthwhile investment, because for little money one can experience good feelings one's whole life. Besides, one can read at any age, whereas other hobbies and interests have to be set aside when one grows older and less energetic.

6.6. Indoor games

Historical records tell us that men have played games from the earliest times. Young children love playing; it gives them a lot of enjoyment. Thousands of different kinds of games are known. Some require physical skills, others intellectual ones, while others are a combination. Games change according to fashion; some die out and new ones take their place. Some games are one person against one; others, one team against another team, but the essential element is competing to win.

Any kind of victory is very exciting and gratifying since it makes us feel good with ourselves and feel admired by others. But the most important factor is not the success, but *being together with others*, usually our friends, doing something thrilling and enjoyable that has no serious repercussions or responsibilities. Another interesting factor is that games are able to erase from our minds and hearts any worries, problems and pains at least during the time the game lasts. For these reasons, games will always be present in our lives as a means of rest.

Some games are highly recommended for older people, as they require a certain intellectual effort which involves keeping to rules and making them. The result of this effort helps to make winning more enjoyable. Examples of games like this are chess, dominoes, draughts and many card games. These indoor games can be played throughout one's life even when one is sick. They have a very positive effect on older people who tend to have negative thoughts and get depressed since one's head is thereby involved in something that does not cause worry or suffering.

Games are a wonderful way to rest from problems and the responsibilities of daily life, and help to keep our minds alert without suffering the tension proper to other kinds of intellectual work since the enjoyment cancels out the tension of the intellectual effort the game entails.

One problem of games, however, is the possibility of becoming addicted and *abandoning one's obligations*, which produces feelings of guilt and failure for not having stopped in time and for having played when one should be doing other things. Therefore, so as not leave a bitter taste, it is advisable to keep strictly to the time one sets aside for games. Together with the addiction one can lose large sums of money. To rest properly it is important to look for *games that one enjoys* and not as a means of earning one's living because the fear of losing money can create much tension.

6.7. Excursions and journeys

As I have said already, our usual daily stimuli constantly remind us of our duties and, without our being aware of it—as a conditioned reflex–, create tension which wears us out. Hence the importance of getting out of our usual rut from time to time because *physical distance* takes us away psychologically from what makes us tired, and helps induce relaxation and rest.

Because of their work, some people have to change environment: go into the street to do their business or travel from one town to another. But as their reason is to achieve objectives they do not relax; they continue working mentally and experience the emotional tension of not knowing the outcomes of their business. But when someone "goes out to enjoy himself" he makes sure his mind will "switch off" from his work and ordinary responsibilities. Thus, he achieves both *physical and psychological "distance"*, and being removed from the "firing line" of ordinary work his head does not "burn" or "freeze"—he avoids exhaustion–, and so he manages to rest.

Excursions and journeys imply enjoyment, and so one tries one's best to achieve this by not talking or thinking of unpleasant things, and immersing oneself fully in these new situations, sights and activities that relax and give pleasure. Therefore, when taking a walk and one comes across people working, *one should not get involved*, so as not to be infected by the atmosphere of tension of the people doing their ordinary duties. Better to adopt an attitude of "lounging", of psychological distance, and so as to not feel indifferent or uncaring keep telling oneself that one is in a holiday mood and out to rest.

Many people go on outings or journeys to see the beauties of nature or art. *Beauty, like goodness, produces a very beneficial psychological effect* since it prompts feelings of peace, serenity and relief, neutralizing any tension or worries. We often make excursions with other people who are close to us in some way. Having more time and deeper interior peace we can get to know them better and mutual affection grows which gives us much joy and even greater energy. Friendship is the best balm for any negative psychological situation and a very effective aid to rest.

One positive thing about journeys and excursions is that whatever one sets out to do are things we like and can release us from the tension caused by duties and responsibilities. We are filled with peace of mind and the happiness that goes with enjoying good and beautiful things.

Lastly, another favourable aspect of this activity is the absence of hurry to do things, which makes it easy to relax. If the outing lasts several days or even weeks, we can relax thoroughly and get rid of all the tension and stress accumulated over time and so feel rested and renew our energy for weeks or months.

6.8. Contemplation

I have often said that to maintain our mental health and joy of living we have to achieve *a balance between the negative and positive aspects of our psychological life*. We must take the poison with its cure which, in terms of health, is like saying tension calls for relaxation, tiredness calls for rest, loneliness for company and suffering for enjoyment, etc.

Now I am going to focus on contemplation or reflection, which is an *antidote to activism* or hustle and bustle, common causes of exhaustion. Activity is tiring, contemplation is restful. Most restful is the contemplation of things that are good, beautiful and true, as I have said in the previous section.

We live in the age of the speed train, which can take us where we want to go extremely fast to do our business. But the speed train does not allow us to see the countryside, and if we try to catch details we are likely to get travel sickness. By shortening journeys there is no longer time to reflect on things as happened in the past when travelling from place to place took several hours.

To rest well, it is recommended to practice *contemplating good things* through the external and internal senses (memory and imagination). To contemplate is to entertain oneself, to savour, to fix one's attention, to immerse oneself in what one is contemplating or let oneself be carried away emotionally by it. Watching children at play; being with someone we like, looking at him and speaking with him; looking at a beautiful landscape; watching and listening to the movement of the sea; listening to beautiful music; feeling the soft touch of a material or fabric; recalling an enjoyable conversation or the affection of someone; tasting and enjoying a good wine; admiring a work of art… These are just some examples of contemplation that give us peace and happiness, help us rest and relax.

Different techniques of meditation could also be mentioned, which are also a kind of mental contemplation of topics that are important for every human being, as well as certain techniques of relaxation where one seeks to reflect on bodily sensations and scenes from our imagination that help us relax. These techniques mean ceasing any activity that is directed towards performance or efficiency, since these consume one's energies.

Obviously, the busiest people and those most committed to fulfilling their obligations convince themselves that they do not have time for reflection and pleasant recreation, but *they are the ones who need it most* so as not to wear themselves out. They must try it out sometime; then they will realize that it does not stop them fulfilling their obligations but helps them do them better and for much longer time.

6.9. Family and friends

The normal thing is that family members and our friends appreciate us and love us the most, though, unfortunately, this is not always the case.

When we are with *people who love us and we feel their love* (it can also happen that they love us but we do not feel loved, because we are closed in ourselves, our worries, sorrows and sufferings), we feel secure and relaxed, because we do not have "to put on an act" to win their love. The confidence we feel when we know they love us and accept us as we are helps us act and speak freely, and releases us from the tension needed to give an acceptable image of ourselves. This way of acting can tire us out. Besides, when one feels loved he has positive feelings: security, joy, and optimism that neutralize the negative ones that accompany tiredness.

It can happen that the reason we get together with friends and relatives is to do things we like (meals, family celebrations, etc.) which we enjoy more and help us rest much more *because of the favorable atmosphere that mutual affection creates.* Hence these family gatherings should not be misused by airing problems or trying to settle quarrels or solve misunderstandings; this can spoil the pleasant atmosphere and ruin its beneficial effects. Unpleasant situations can arise more easily if too much alcohol and other substances are consumed because they reduce self-control and increase susceptibilities and the possibility of misunderstandings.

When one is especially tired it is good to remember the restorative and beneficial effect of seeking out loved ones and enjoying their company. But it is even better to meet them regularly to prevent such bouts of tiredness altogether. Therefore, it is advisable to *get used to being with family members and friends* at fixed times, not only birthdays and other celebrations, but also just to take a coffee or drink a beer, go shopping or do sports together, or just to chat.

6.10 Hunting, fishing and other outdoor activities

Contact with nature and gathering its fruits is something natural to man; originally as a means of survival, but nowadays mainly to enjoy oneself.

This activity has several attractive ingredients and is a wonderful means of rest. First, there is the beauty and peacefulness of nature, which gives us much relief. Then, the pleasure in finding the fruits of nature we are looking for, such as animals, fishes, mushrooms, wild fruits, butterflies, flowers, birds, etc. Our whole attention is centred on the search and so we forget our worries and problems, and the tension they produce. The *happiness of looking for things and finding them* cancels out the negative feelings of daily life. And as we usually go there with friends or relatives, we all have a good time together.

There are many things to be found in nature, and everyone can find something that will give him pleasure, always provided we respect the environment, especially by not dropping litter where we go. One can go to the countryside, to a mountain or the sea to look for and experience beautiful landscapes, pleasant sounds like the singing of birds, the roar of the ocean or streams and waterfalls, the smell of plants and flowers, of wet grass, burnt wood, or the taste of fruits growing in the wild.

People who live stressed lives in big cities can gain a lot from these. In addition there is the physical exercise involved, which is very good for people who are seated most of the day; the important thing is to try to be constant and regular.

6.11. Laughter and good humour

From time to time in the various media we can read an article on the healthy benefits of laughter and good humour. There is some truth in this but alone they are not the panacea to physical and psychological health.

Because of the psychosomatic unity of mind and body, physical events and facts can affect our psychological functions and vice versa. Laughter, which is something physical, produces psychological changes like the *appearance of positive feelings*, happiness, relaxation, and optimism. The more often and longer we laugh the deeper and more lasting are the positive feelings, and, as a consequence, the deeper the relief from the negative feelings that go with tiredness.

The muscles that tense with laughter are many more than those that tense when we smile. Besides, they react with the muscles that tighten when we are stressed or tense. From Newton's law of "action and reaction", when one muscles contracts its opposite relaxes. Hence the effect of relaxation and physical rest which produces laughter. I have often said that to rest we have to enjoy ourselves, so *when we laugh we are in full enjoyment.*

It is very restful to *take part in things that make us laugh a lot.* Some are readily available, such as watching comedies, funny videos especially on Internet, listening to someone who tells jokes well, remembering amusing incidents with others, playing decent jokes on others, etc.

Practising laughing at funny things can make it easier to *laugh at ourselves* and not take ourselves too seriously. Some people take themselves too seriously and always feel tense and exhausted. This can help us not to dramatize everything that happens in life, the only life we have, and learn to look on the bright side.

Being always good-humoured is an excellent way to *prevent chronic stress* and psychological exhaustion. For those around us it is a balm of peace and joy that will help them rest too. It also creates an atmosphere of calm that infects others. To achieve this it helps to surround oneself with cheerful and amusing people and avoid the sad, worried or bitter types. Nor should one spoil a pleasant atmosphere with accounts of negative events or with discussions that are out of place or stupid. Amusing moments are to be enjoyed and sad ones to suffer. We should try to have more of the first and fewer of the others, and not mix them.

6.12 Manual skills and repairs

In recent years with the increasing popularity of do-it-yourself people are now starting to install their own furniture (a well-known Swedish multi-national has made it very easy), and to do their own house repairs and make many gadgets for leisure (modelling, marquetry, etc.).

When we try to do *manual activities* very well and feel happy with what we have done, and for others to like them too, we focus all our attention on what we are doing and forget the worries, duties and responsibilities of every day; we rest in them. The more we apply ourselves to manual skills and the more time we devote to them the more profound will be our rest from ordinary tasks.

These manual tasks help those people to rest who have *some talent in this area,* but clumsy people suffer because they do not know how to do them or they do them badly and so feel they have wasted their time. In addition they get annoyed and feel frustrated and discouraged when other reproach them telling them what they have done is useless. Such negative feelings do not make it easy for them to rest; instead they add to the tiredness they had before they began the work. People without manual skills need to find other activities to help them rest. Each wayfarer follows his own path and each man his own way of resting.

However, there are some manual jobs that less skilled people can do well, like simple repairs: changing a light-bulb, mowing the lawn, putting order in the store, jigsaw puzzles, Sudoku, knitting, making bracelets, necklaces, etc.

The idea is to rest from intellectual work by doing manual tasks and vice-versa: rest from physical tiredness with activities that involve the mind, such as reading, music, art, and history. This is in line with the final objective: equilibrium of work and rest, the physical and the intellectual in this case.

6.13 Gardening and horticulture

Caring for the garden, the terrace, the flower-pots on the balcony and the vegetable garden are also manual skills, but with one small difference, in that they allow us to gather the fruits. Gardening and plants reward us with the beauty of nature enclosed in a garden patch and some flower-pots. In the case of the vegetable garden, besides the beauty of the plants when they are in season we gather their fruits which we can taste, and smell their true aroma, unaffected by processes to preserve them. There is nothing quite like eating straight from a tree or a vegetable patch. And so, besides enjoying the physical exercise and the manual work, the visual beauty of a garden full of plants and fruit trees, we have the satisfaction of being "creators" (like a painter at his easel) and providers of pleasure to those who eat from the work of our hands.

The natural feeling man has to be close to nature and enjoy its goodness has given rise to something widespread throughout the world: a small house in the country-side, with a patch of land to grow vegetables and to retire there, on a weekend or a holiday and rest in natural surroundings.

Contact with the land is very satisfying since nature is good and appreciative. If we treat her well, she will treat us well in return, reward us with pleasant feelings and raise our spirits and relieve us of the fatigue of daily life.

It is often said that the good and the bad thrive together everywhere. But my impression, although not based on statistics, is that the most balanced, healthy and sound people—at least the ones I know—are in contact with nature in one way or another.

6.14 Mascots and pets

I have already said that one way of feeling good and resting is to be with people who like us and whom we like. This applies also to *being with things we like*, such as interests and hobbies. Liking and loving always produce positive feelings and emotions, which cancel out the negative ones that go with tiredness.

Mutatis mutandis (with due alteration of details comparing two cases), the same happens when one is with animals that one likes and by which we feel liked. To look after these creatures, play with them and receive their affection is so pleasant as to capture our attention and make us forget our worries, problems and frustrations. It helps us rest, because love is the best medicine for suffering and fatigue.

On the other hand, to show our concern for them makes us feel good with ourselves, as a consequence of giving ourselves and helping, so that we neutralize the negative feelings of tiredness and we rest from our usual routine.

6.15 Prayer and spiritual activities

On a completely different level we have prayer and religious activities. Not everyone has religious sensibility, but many find calm, peace of mind and rest when they address a Superior Being whom they think of as Creator of the universe and loving Father who wants the best for his children. And if He, who is almighty, "rested" from his work of creating the universe and wanted this to be recorded in the Bible for us to know, we too should rest after doing our work.

In the peace of a church, leaving the hustle and bustle of life outside, it is easy to recover our calm and feel more relaxed. Besides, one feels a great relief and rest when considering the burdens of life and the fatigue of one's problems before the glance of the Almighty, who is our Father who loves us and, therefore, *is ready to help us solve our problems or give us strength to bear them.* Thus, to pray or meditate frequently in the presence of God can help us rest without becoming worn out.

Often in the presence of God we see problems and duties in a different light, as they really are, and less important than we think and so they weigh us down less and we do not feel so tired.

Also, when we speak to God about what burdens us and tires us, it can be helpful to accept it and so we understand that we can offer it as a sacrifice to ask pardon for our sins and those of other people as a means of penance for the offences against God. By accepting this "burden" we feel less tired and more relieved. "When there is a why the how doesn't matter". If we have a good reason for suffering and feeling tired the intensity of the effort involved is not so important and the burden feels lighter.

Speaking with God (prayer) also helps us to rest because it enables us to *unburden ourselves* with Him and feel his presence in our tiredness. Whenever we share the psychological burden of ordinary worries they feel less oppressive and one does not get so tired.

EPILOGUE

Some people are so committed to being successful in this life or are moved by an excessive sense of duty that they forget that we are in this world to be happy and help others to be happy. An unhappy person cannot teach others to be happy.

It is true that one element needed for happiness is to do things well, and our conscience will tell us what things we must do and how we must do them. But, to be happy we also need to *feel free*. That is, *we must do what we have to do and do it well, but with a free spirit because "we feel like doing it"*. When we do things because we are afraid of failing or suffering, feeling guilty or useless, then we do not act freely or freely enough because our fear, which is something of the emotions, limits our freedom.

It is true that our emotions accompany all we do in life, but we have to learn to control them and train them so that instead of being a hindrance to freedom they strengthen our will-power and help us to be more free and therefore more happy.

In our task of attaining an equilibrium, in which the higher power must control the lower, between the head (intelligence and will) and the affectivity (feelings, emotions, states of mind) the normal process of *psychological maturation* plays a role to favour mental health and help us be happy. The contrary (disequilibrium) produces immature personalities (pathologically neurotic) condemned to suffer a certain degree of anguish, and who will not find happiness easily.

Many of the people who suffer anxiety are in a permanent state of psychological tension. This leads to the debilitation of vital energies ending in physical exhaustion and psychological illness. Until they achieve psychological maturity, which is the work of a lifetime, they must find an adequate balance between the negative and the positive: tiredness and rest, duty and devotion, suffering and enjoyment, activity and restfulness, tension and relaxation, company and solitude, sleep and wakefulness. Only in this way can they prevent exhaustion.

When the disequilibrium is very pronounced, or less pronounced but lasts for a long time, it ends with a physical and/or psychological breakdown. Some sooner, others later, depending on one's psychological resistance and age. Hence the importance of prevention, and of realizing this oneself or being warned in good time.

Prevention is always better than cure. Therefore, it is essential to understand that together with one's duties in the outside world, the more important task is take care of one's interior world, which is to manage to have and to maintain one's joy and peace of mind, despite everything else. This is how we can avoid chronic exhaustion and bouts of tiredness which make it hard to lead a happy life and to make our loved ones happy, because these are much more important than all material possessions.

BIBLIOGRAPHY

CABANYES, J. y MONGE, M. Á. (eds.), *La salud mental y sus cuidados,* 2nd. ed., EUNSA, Pamplona 2010. A very useful resource to expound on some of the topics I have dealt with in my book. The study by GAMAO GARRÁN, P., *El estrés en la vida cotidiana,* 253-264, is the most directly connected to rest and it has a robust bibliography.

LECLERCQ, J. y PIEPER, J., *De la vida serena,* Rialp, Madrid 1965. The reader will find in this small book, which contains a magisterial write up by each author, very suggestive reflections about the basic and importance of serenity.

MARTÍ GARCÍA, M. Á., *La serenidad. Una actitud ante el mundo,* 3th. ed., Ediciones Internacionales Universitarias, Madrid 2005.
—*El sosiego. Una filosofía de vida,* Ediciones Internacionales Universitarias, Madrid 2007.

PHILIPPE, J., *Interior Freedom.*, Rialp, Madrid 2007.

PIEPER, J., *El ocio y la vida intelectual,* Rialp, Madrid 1983.
—*Una teoría de la fiesta,* Rialp, Madrid 1974.

SILES SALINAS, J., *El ocio la contemplación, la intimidad,* Atlántida, Madrid 1970, 362-386.

VV.AA., Voz "Descanso", en *Gran Enciclopedia Rialp,* tomo VII, Madrid 1992, 562-567. This entry contains various articles that deal with rest from various perspectives: medical, biblical and ethical.

YEPES, R., *La región de lo lúdico: Reflexión sobre el fin y la forma del juego,* en Cuadernos de Anuario Filosófico, n. 30, Servicio de Publicaciones de la Universidad de Navarra Pamplona 1996.

Further reading

- Interior freedom by Jacques Philippe.
- Leisure, the basis of culture by Josef Pieper

ABOUT THE AUTHOR

Fernando Sarráis was born in Mérida, Spain, in 1958. He graduated in Medicine and Surgery in the University of the Basque Country and obtained a doctorate in Medicine and Surgery from the University of Navarre. He has a degree in Psychology from the Spanish National University of Distance Learning. He has been specialist in psychiatry since 1998. He is currently an Associate Professor of the Psychopathy of Education and Social Psychology in the University of Navarre.

Other books by this author

- El árbol de la vida (mental), cuyo fruto es la Felicidad
- 30 consejos para una vida feliz
- Familia en armonía
- El diálogo
- Entender la afectividad
- Psicopatologia
- Temperamento, carácter y personalidad
- Personalidad
- Análisis psicológico del hombre
- Madurez psicológica y felicidad
- Temas de psicología práctica
- El miedo
- Afectividad y sexualidad

Find more at fernandosarrais.com

www.ingramcontent.com/pod-product-compliance
Ingram Content Group UK Ltd.
Pitfield, Milton Keynes, MK11 3LW, UK
UKHW022011190726
13853UKWH00004B/1872